WE GOT THIS!

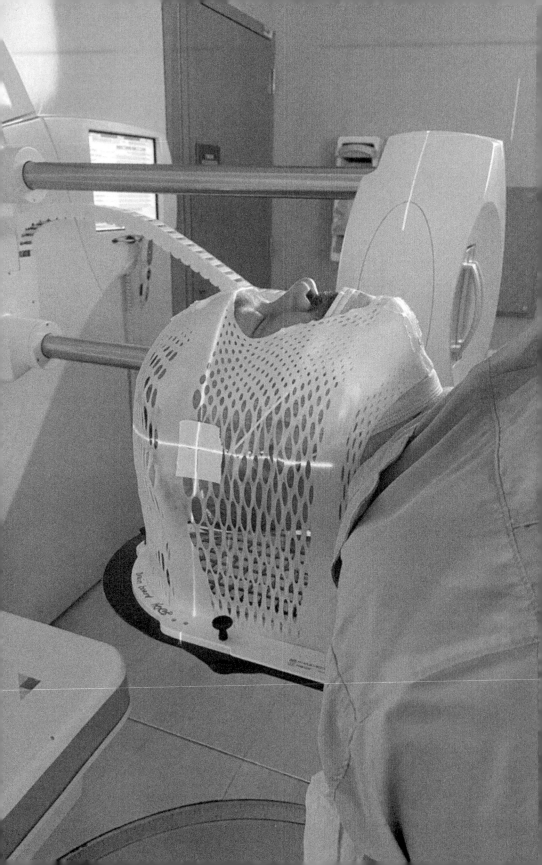

LEADERSHIP PRINCIPLES
LEARNED & REINFORCED
THROUGH A 12-MONTH BATTLE WITH CANCER

JIMMY KITSON

BMD Publishing

WE GOT THIS!
Leadership Principles Learned & Reinforced
Through a 12-Month Battle with Cancer

Copyright © 2022 Jimmy Kitson

BMD Publishing
All Rights Reserved

ISBN # 979-8423188313

BMDPublishing@MarketDominationLLC.com
www.MarketDominationLLC.com

BMD Publishing CEO: Seth Greene
Editorial Management: Bruce Corris
Technical Editor & Layout: Kristin Watt

Printed in the United States of America.

Dedicated to Christy, Connor, and Kelcie

CONTENTS

FOREWORD

It was a sunny spring day in 2005 when I first met Jimmy Kitson. I was 18 months out of college, dressed in my best on-sale suit from The Limited, slightly scuffed heels from Nine West, and my beloved pink sparkle Motorola Razr flip phone in my purse. Our group of new hires met Jimmy on the first day where he stood at the front of the classroom. Tall, bald, and serious.

During those two weeks 17 years ago, through his support, challenge, and unwavering commitment to developing others, Jimmy laid down what was to be the foundation of my career within medical device sales. Like myself, so many have had the benefit of Jimmy's leadership and his desire to help others grow.

As you'll learn through his story, in 2021, Jimmy went through one of life's greatest challenges, the fight for his life. When this happened, people came out in droves to support him.

Among the many words of appreciation and thanks to this amazing leader were comments like "I wouldn't be here if it wasn't for Jimmy," "Jimmy hired me when no one else would," "Jimmy was the best boss I've ever worked for," and "There is nothing I wouldn't do for Jimmy...he did everything for me."

You're reading this book for a very important reason. It means you are someone who wants more for those around you. You are a person who is inspired by leading and developing others, and I'm here to tell you, you picked the right story.

You'll walk away with many life and leadership lessons that will have you asking yourself daily... "Is this my best work?" If the answer is "yes" then Jimmy has done his job...for we are a reflection of him, our success is his success and our achievements happened because he cared. Because he led. Because he leaned in and saw something in us that at the time, we didn't see in ourselves. Because he helped us go from good to great and be our best selves.

So, Jimmy, when you sit back and reflect on all those you've made an impact on, know that the list is long and your impact monumental. Know that we carry you in our hearts and we wouldn't be the leaders we are today without your influence on our lives.

We are truly better because of you. Starting with Christy, Connor, and Kelcie and spanning far and wide....my dear friend...we are your best work.

-Leigh Spellman

ACKNOWLEDGMENTS

There have been a ton of people to support us throughout this fight against cancer. Thank you to all the following groups and individuals.

1. I have worked with two remarkable companies over the last 20 years of my career. First, Smith & Nephew. The support from the Smith & Nephew team in helping us determine best places to get supplies and help coordinate calls with other key wound care physicians was excellent. They even came to our home during a complex dressing change to teach the home nurse and my wife the best way to apply the dressings. That was greatly appreciated. And your gift to our family brought us such optimism and joy. Special Thanks to LA, RV, LS, EH, MF and TS for going beyond the normal call of duty. We are feeding the Courage Wolf!

2. The company I currently work for, Align Technology, has shown my family and me what it is like to truly support an employee. Every interaction I have had with leadership since my cancer diagnosis has always been about my health. They have never tried to rush me back

into work, reinforcing the culture we talk about in the meetings about respecting each individual, and working through our corporate values focusing on accountability, customer, and agility. I hope we did not ask for much during my time away, but everything we ever needed, including the Month of Smiles gesture, was greatly cherished. Special thanks to MM, TJ, NM, JG, M-UM, AS, and MN.

3. We could not have gotten through 2021 without the support of my NC State fraternity brothers, especially Matt, Doug, Pat, Jason, and Johnny. The help provided by many of the friends we have met in Texas, Wisconsin, and our home in NC over the years was astonishing. The text messages or phone calls to me always came at the right time when the challenges were getting bigger and more complex. The meals and desserts, letting our dogs out when we were running behind from an appointment or event, the carpool help for our daughter, and the personalized gifts sent to us were definitely unexpected but were timely to receive. These were huge time-savers as we rushed from hospital to hospital, worked around crazy radiation schedules and wound care treatments, and managed through physical therapy. Special thanks to the McClendons, Gilberts, Dumonts, Coynes, Newmans, Knoxes, Sanderses, and both Smith families (Jason & Sherrie and Eric & Carolyn). You all are so special to us.

4. Thank you to all of the nurses and doctors who treated us in all sorts of care settings, both at MUSC in Charleston and UNC–Chapel Hill. Words cannot express how lucky I was to be cared for by each one of you. A special Thank You to Amy, David, Terry, Josh, Hannah, and Sara.

5. To The Foo Fighters and the casts of Ted Lasso and Yellowstone. Every surgical procedure and every 30-minute radiation treatment had the Foo Fighters cranking as I went in. Friday nights were "Date Night" for Christy and me as we watched Ted Lasso, which is probably the best comedy and inspirational TV show we have seen. Once Ted Lasso concluded, Date Night switched to Sunday night for Yellowstone. Thank you for being there for us.

6. To my mom, Mike, Josh, Suzanne, Jamie, Mary, Matthew, Jessie, Courtney, and Patrick - I appreciate the love that you have shown us and dropping all things in your world to help keep our world afloat. We could not have done it without you.

7. To my children, Connor and Kelcie – I am so proud of the strength you have shown these last 18 months, dealing with Covid issues and then my cancer diagnosis. This was unfair to you, and yet you still excelled as students, athletes, making good decisions and being positive humans. When I was growing up and people asked me what I wanted to be, I many times told them I just wanted to be a good dad, which I strive for every

day with you. I love you both so much and am blessed and proud to call you my children.

8. Finally, to my wife, Christy. On our second date, I told you I was going to marry you, and here we are, 21 years later battling through this. You handled the last eight months of 2021 with grace, compassion, and empathy. You have become an expert in setting up group texts to notify everyone how I was doing. You should be awarded an honorary nursing degree for your proficiency in changing wound dressings. There is a special place in heaven reserved for people like you. My universe has always and will always revolve around you first, because that is what makes me happy. You have shown me what true and selfless love is and I am in awe of you. I love you.

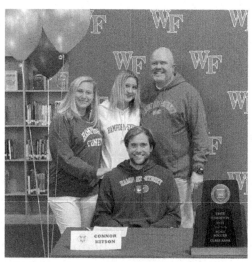

Connor's College Signing Day.
This photo was taken days before my cancer surgery.

A NOTE TO THE READER

For years, many of my friends have been trying to get me to write a book on leadership. I have been a leader for over 20 years, for teams of four up to more than 100. I have made mistakes, learned from them, and hopefully imparted some wisdom onto those I have led and worked alongside. One of the goals I shared with a new person who worked for me was this: "10 years from now, when you are asked who had the biggest impact on you and your leadership style and inspired you to do your best in a fair and ethical manner, I want to be that answer". I knew I would never have close to 100% of the people list me as their influencer, but I have many people who call to talk to me when asked that question by others, whether it is in an interview or development class.

Originally, I wanted to be the type of leader that I would have liked to work for. But I quickly learned that while that was great for someone similar to my personality and emotional intelligence traits, it did not work for everyone. I received a DiSC Personality certification, truly immersed myself into this concept to understand what others needed and to make sure I was leading my teams the way they needed to be led, not how I wanted to lead.

I chose to start a blog (www.alwayslearningleader.com) seven years ago as I did not have the time or energy to concentrate on a book. My friend Michael Niezgoda told me when he learned of my cancer diagnosis in early 2021 that while this cancer news sucked, this was a defining event. I had to write a book to hopefully inspire others diagnosed with cancer and to share my story of healing, because we all knew we were going to defy the odds and beat this thing. My wife agreed with Michael and this is our journey.

Let me point out a couple things about the way this book is written. First, it was entirely written by me. No ghost writer. This is my story, and these are my words. But it is not always written from my perspective. I use both "I" and we, along with "mine" and "ours". If any of my former English teachers are reading this, I apologize for the fits that may cause you. This grammar decision is intentional and purposeful. We wanted to share this experience as we fought it, as a team. While my mind and body had to personally fight and overcome all these health struggles, it was always a team effort to get through a surgery, or survive a nasty infection or seizure. I could never have fought this battle alone and this is what we are trying to share by shifting the point of view throughout the book.

Each chapter begins with a timeframe of the events for that chapter. At the end of each chapter, we will also include a QR Code and link to take you to a site that will have color pictures from each time period and will be updated regularly as we continue our pathway to healing.

Please note, these pictures are real. Some are graphic. We are sharing them with you because they chronicle what we went through.

This is our journey...

PROLOGUE

*JANUARY 2021

In writing out my goals for the year in January 2021, I was brought back to a saying that I had heard years ago from someone who was getting ready to hit a milestone - their 50th birthday. They said, "I want my 50s to be better than my 40s". I took this slogan to heart and copied it as I was documenting some personal goals along with my professional goals for work. I always had hand-written goals because I felt the goal meant more when it was written in my own handwriting versus printed in Garamond, Times New Roman, or Arial font. The year 2021 had to be better than 2020 with Covid, the political climate of our country, and the social injustices that many felt and personally endured all negatively headlining the news in 2020. It was time to move forward in many ways.

I am a lucky man. I have an incredible wife, Christy, and two wonderful children, Connor and Kelcie. We also have two dogs (Honey and Daisy) that Kelcie made me mention in the book as they too are part of our family. We have lived in Wake Forest, NC since 2013. We enjoy the weather and seasonal changes NC offers, and we love being so close to both the beach and mountains.

I have worked in a variety of positions with two medical companies, Smith and Nephew and currently with Align Technology, more widely known as the maker of Invisalign. My current role is wonderful and rewarding. I have the privilege of working with our Align Faculty members to educate other doctors and offices to help "Transform Smiles and Change Lives". I get to work across many different segments to help educate the industry on why our clinically dominant product and portfolio should be used on every appropriate patient. I have never worked with a group of faculty or speakers who are more passionate about a brand and willing to spend many hours teaching others. It is a great partnership and I appreciate all of them and their work.

My passions outside work are two-fold. First is my passion for soccer. Both my kids play. They love it and fortunately are pretty good at the sport...much better than I was at their ages. My wife and I try to attend every game for both of them (a little more difficult with Connor now playing in college in Virginia), and we greet them after every game with "I love watching you play". Win, lose, or draw, this is the conversation starter when we first see them. I have seen too many parents berate their kids during and after a game and promised myself I would never do that to our children. I am also on the board of directors for NCFC Youth Soccer, which is one of the largest youth soccer clubs in the U.S. I have led the U10 Boys Challenge League for eight seasons and love supporting the volunteer coaches with their players. Our board is an incredibly talented group, and the positive momentum that Gary Buete and his team have built since he arrived will only continue. I love to give back to the sport I enjoyed playing while in grade school and college, and loved watching any time a game is on TV. YNWA!!!

My other passion is cooking and specifically using my Traeger smoker to cook pulled pork, ribs, and anything else that could use a kiss of pecan wood smoke. BBQ is something that almost always unites but occasionally divides (Eastern NC sauce vs Western NC sauce, pulled pork vs beef brisket, etc.). There is nothing better than starting the smoker at midnight, putting on a couple of pork shoulders, and pulling them off 15 hours later. The smell permeates our neighborhood and it seems like our neighbors magically appear to say hi and see what our dinner plans are. BBQ brings people together and we love to cook it, share it, and eat it.

When we lived in Texas, we had a hard time finding good NC pulled pork, as Texas is more known for brisket and ribs. One day in 2011, I told Christy that I was going to make my own rub and sauce and we would just improvise to get that NC flavor into the food we cooked in our backyard. We experimented with a couple different versions of a sauce and rub. I would bring bottles of sauce and sandwich bags filled with spices into our Smith and Nephew offices in Fort Worth, where we had a number of good grill masters to test and give us feedback. After finalizing the recipes which would yield

20 jars of rub and six bottles of sauce per batch, Connor asked "What are we going to call this?" I told him we would call it the Bald Man Rub (for good luck) for the spice, and Bald Man Mop Sauce for the sauce. He then proceeded to make our first label, the bottle of which we still have now.

BBQ is a great hobby. We love to cook and support others. We would make batches of rub and sauce in our kitchen around Thanksgiving and Christmas to share with friends and family as gifts. We used this product to cook at different charity events throughout the years, never asking for payment. We felt so good about the mouths we fed at a charity we supported or at the firehouses that protected us. We were actually being asked where these guests could buy the rub and sauce. We all laughed at the thought of making enough out of our kitchen for stores. But in 2018, Connor and I spent a couple months researching manufacturing, marketing, and how to sell our product to local stores. We met a marvelous partner, Karen, who came up with our slogan "Good Better Bald" and helped us with branding and website building. In 2019, Bald Man BBQ started and we began shipping out product to local shops and online. We have been asked to get into bigger stores, but that was never the purpose of this project. We just want to make some people happy and eat some good food. BBQ became our fifth priority, behind Family, Faith, Work and Soccer.

Prior to 2021, I can tell you that I was truly blessed (and still am from a different perspective). We could travel when we wanted (pre-Covid), we loved to hang out with family and friends, and we were all healthy.

That is, until January of 2021.

I am going to share some very brief parts of our cancer journey with you in this book and each chapter will conclude with a leadership principle from this story and how it can make you a better spouse, parent, child, employee, or leader. The great NC State coach Jimmy Valvano said, "If you laugh, you think, and you cry, that's a full day. That's a heck of a day. You do that seven days a week, you're going to have something special."

I hope this book gets you to do one of those three.

CHAPTER 1

The New Normal

*JANUARY 2021 – MARCH 2021

As 2020 was coming to a close and people geared up for a more positive 2021, the term "New Normal" was introduced to our world. We would never be the same as we were prior to Covid, but optimism was high for many heading into the year. For the Kitson family, Connor was getting ready to start his last semester of high school and trying to defend their state soccer championship title from the previous season (they wound up losing in the final eight). College visits were tough because of visitation rules and Covid concerns, but he had multiple offers to attend a college and play soccer, or just be a college student and enjoy life. Kelcie was enjoying getting back to in-person school even though it was only a couple days per week. She loves being with her friends and playing soccer, and like many others, the last eight months of 2020 into the spring semester of 2021 were not a fun time for her and her middle school friends.

Christy and I were getting our stuff together to close out 2020, and move into 2021. She had another successful year as a realtor and had a good first quarter lined up. I was ready to get back to live in-person programs for our customers. Zoom calls had helped us all stay connected while we had curfews and stay-at-home mandates, but I am a people person (High I for the DiSC people). While I enjoyed seeing everyone's faces virtually each day, spending eight hours a day on Zoom calls was becoming more taxing to endure.

In mid-January, I noticed two bumps on the top of my head. This was not too much of a cause for concern as I have had many of these similar types of areas removed over the years. From Lipoma tumors to basal cells, my head, arms, legs and back all had scars from many excisions or Mohs surgeries. Growing up near the beach and living on a horse farm, my body was constantly in the sun. I tanned pretty quickly, so I avoided the typical sunburns felt by my sisters and brother. I hardly wore sunscreen until after college. However, we now know a lot more about the effects of sun on the skin and needless to say my children have been properly bathed in SPF 50 sunscreen since birth. I was also awaiting my annual check-up in March, which was a big one as I was turning 50. I wanted my bloodwork and other vitals to have improved since I was 45, and was feeling pretty good, exercising, and eating as well as a carnivore can eat. I literally eat nothing green.

One new area of concern with these bumps on the top of my head was that I was experiencing headaches. Not the migraine type of headaches, but ones that would last for five to six hours and be at a pain level of five out of 10 (One out of 10 is no pain and 10 out of 10 is excruciating). I attributed the headaches to my many Zoom calls, and knew that getting back into the office live and in person was going to help these go away. In February, I started going back into the office a day or two a week to just get away from my office in our home.

I had my check-up appointment with our primary care physician, Dr. Amy Shipley, on March 9th. I told her about the headaches and showed her the bumps on my head and she told me to get a CT scan just to make sure they were not problematic. My weight had decreased each year over the last five years, my bloodwork all came back in normal levels, and I was feeling really good about the visit after reviewing this information with her. I was a pretty healthy 50-year-old man regarding my vitals and annual checkup.

I had my CT scan late on Thursday that week as it was a busy week of meetings and programs at night. I received a call from Dr. Shipley on Friday morning that would change the rest of my life. She said that the CT scan had revealed some troublesome signs and I needed to schedule an MRI immediately. I told her the next two weeks were pretty busy with work, my birthday, and soccer for the kids. She countered, "Jimmy you need this done Monday or Tuesday next week".

I went in for the MRI on the morning of my birthday at UNC Hospital's Imaging Center at 6:45am. I was the first one there and the office was eerily quiet. I checked in with the receptionist and was told to wait back in the car until the MRI machine turned on at 7:00am. They called me back five minutes later. I undressed and put on a robe, the nurse inserted an IV into my arm, and I was led to the room with the MRI machine, where I would spend the next 60 minutes laying on a flat board with my head secured in place. Certain people can handle things, like enclosed MRI tubes, better than others. I have never been scared of tight or enclosed areas like MRI or CT scan machines. I close my eyes once entering the tube, focus on breathing slowly, and try to understand the thumping and rhythms of the insanely loud machine. Once the scans were completed, I drove the 45 minutes home in silence. I was hopeful they would find nothing but in the back of my mind, I was prepared for the worst. Christy and I had kept these scans and appointments very private, not even telling our kids.

On the way home, I received a call from Dr. Shipley. I had a very large tumor growing in my head. They were not aware of what type of cancer it was or the extent of the damage. However, there was major concern that the tumor was growing into the dura layer of my brain (not good) and had impacted the area around the sagittal sinus vein in my head (even worse). I needed to get back to UNC within the next 24 hours to have surgical biopsies performed to try and determine the type of cancer. I told Christy when I got home. We both had a ton of questions that we wrote down, and we cried, hugged, and cried some more. We told our kids that day at lunch as they were still home with virtual school. Connor was a rock and told us, "We Got This," which would soon become our rallying cry. My precious 13-year-old Kelcie fought back tears but then we finally broke down together. Being vulnerable is healthy, crying with your friends, family, and co-workers even more so.

That night we had a great 50th birthday dinner with some of our closest friends. We did not tell our friends as we still had questions and not enough answers. We did our best to enjoy the evening, but it was tough. I feel Christy and I are pretty genuine and authentic people and we were just processing the news from the day and were pretty quiet at dinner. We were not the same people that night. Our friends knew something was up and they would find out soon.

Our new normal was changing...and quickly. Our 2021 would be much more difficult than 2020.

ALWAYS LEARNING LEADER TAKEAWAYS:

The ability to be agile is critical for a leader of any magnitude - a parent, coach, manager, or any other role that you can influence others. Nobody sets a plan for failure, yet there are many teams and organizations that do not hit their objective. The first two months of 2021 were business as usual for us, professionally and personally. Everything was great and we were continuing to live our best life. However, we got hit with this devastating blow in March. The month of April would set the tone for the rest of the year. Our New Normal would change drastically from our original goal sheet filled out in January. We were knocked down but our comeback was going to be greater than our setback.

- When your plan gets shot down or does not work, fail fast to shift gears to something more beneficial. Start asking questions of what led to the situation going poorly. Was it controllable? In my instance, I did not have a great deal of control other than probably using more sunscreen as a kid. There are several leaders I have worked for in the past who I admire. They always ask the right questions to get your mind working toward a solution. Typically, when we struggled, it was because people did not believe in the purpose or a process was broken. I don't know anyone who wakes up in the morning saying they are going to perform poorly that day.

- When you hear or learn of bad news, don't criticize or berate, but ask questions about what to do moving forward. Focus on the next 30 days to turn around the situation with the right purpose and process in place. We learned this valuable lesson in the first week after hearing of cancer and potential treatments. We were focused on how long it would take to heal completely, what the percentages were for recovery, and how quickly I could get back to work and swing a golf club again. Our doctors calmed us down by telling us that we needed to survive each week to get to the end result. So, I set minor goals, like attending my son's high school graduation in person in June (completed) and being able to take my wife out to an anniversary dinner in August (failed on this one and will share why in future chapters).

VIEW THE PICTURES THAT
CHRONICLE OUR JOURNEY

ALWAYSLEARNINGLEADER.COM/WE-GOT-THIS-PICTURES/

CHAPTER 2

Asking Questions
& Active Listening
*MARCH 2021 – APRIL 2021

The next two weeks had us trying to determine what type of cancer we had and what the options were for treatment. We also had another MRI three weeks after the first one and the tumors were growing quickly. Time was of the essence and we needed surgery and radiation and/or chemo to help get this cancer out of my body.

We had decided to do the surgery at Medical University of South Carolina (MUSC) in Charleston as I had developed some connections there over the years, both personally and professionally. They also were one of the leaders in this type of treatment and planning and we felt very comfortable with them. We would handle any type of post-surgical chemotherapy or radiation at UNC-Chapel Hill as this was closer to home.

The initial surgical biopsy indicated that the tumor was

a basal cell that was somehow growing a lot differently than typical basal cells external from the skin. Mine was unfortunately growing inward. It was pushing on the dura layer of my brain and applying pressure on my brain. When I first met with one of our surgeons and he looked at my head and our scans, he stated, "You should not have this type of cancer and complications at your age. You have been dealt a shit hand." We learned that the average age of someone who has this type of basal cell skin cancer is nearly 70, and the prognosis when it is on your brain is not good. I did not know how to reply so I just listened as they talked about how they were going to treat my case. I had represented some of the best products in wound care for 15 years, and helped clinicians heal wounds that I could have never imagined healing. I knew a ton about wound care, and how hospitals work. Now I was the patient.

Their plan was to have the neurosurgeon start the surgery and take out as much of the tumor as he safely could. Next a team would come in to remove the affected portion of my skull and put a titanium mesh plate in place. Finally, a plastic surgeon would come and REMOVE my left lat muscle from my back to place on my head, and tie in the veins and arteries from my lat to my head. Surgery would take 14 to 18 hours, and I would need 14 days in the hospital to recover. I would then transition home to North Carolina and receive seven weeks of daily radiation in Chapel Hill. We would have a home health nurse visit us four days a week to help with anything wound care or cancer related. I would also have a pretty weirdly shaped head for eight months until things began to heal better. The doctors told us that 20% of patients don't make it out of surgery alive, and I needed to make sure my affairs were in order. What I heard was that 80% of patients survived and I was going to be in the majority.

All of that was a lot to handle in our first meeting with them. But they stressed that time was of the essence and we had a week to prepare for surgery. We had a ton of questions, but I don't think we knew the right questions to ask, and we weren't fully understanding what was happening. In 15 years of being in and out of hospitals and helping patients heal their wounds, I had never seen or heard of a procedure like this. Life was a blur for us. We were just trying to figure out what we were getting into and what our next couple weeks would look like.

We also figured that we needed to disclose the news of my cancer with certain family members and some of our closest friends. After sharing the news, the questions our family and friends were asking us were the ones we needed to ask of our surgeons immediately. Our friends and family, while shocked by what we shared with them, were way more rational in their thinking than we were. We started to ask our doctors the questions we were being asked, and we became way more informed from this process.

There were complications in our immediate family. My daughter had knee surgery the week before my surgery to help heal some torn cartilage. She would be on crutches for a few weeks and have to start physical therapy without us there to help. The day of my surgery was also college signing day for my son at his high school. Christy and I looked at our calendars and realized we needed help and a plan. Meal trains were created. Connor was able to help with basic parenting for Kelcie, and family members also helped by staying at our home with the kids, and helping them with whatever was needed, including getting Kelcie to PT. Coach Joyner and Coach Pittarelli, the Athletic Director and Soccer Coach at Wake Forest High School, graciously moved Connor's signing day to the Friday before the school ceremony, allowing us to attend as they honored Connor and his best friend Jake Smith, the two soccer players moving on to play in college. What a great gesture by these two coaches and the Smith family. The family photo taken of us that day, which you saw at the end of my acknowledgments would be the last picture of me I would post on social media for a while.

On Sunday, two days before surgery, I played nine holes of golf with Connor, and our friend Gary and his son Will. It was great to step away from all of the cancer talk and do something mind-numbing on a warm spring afternoon. When Connor and I got home, Jake and his father Jason were finishing up delivering a La-Z-Boy recliner to our home. Part of recovery was going to require my head staying higher than my body for a while. Christy had bought me a wedge pillow for sleeping in the bed, but we came to find that the recliner was way more comfortable to sleep in when we got home.

Surgery was scheduled for 6:00 am on Tuesday, April 27th. We knew it would be a long day, with surgery lasting up to 18 hours. All sorts of preparatory tasks had to take place the day before the surgery, including a PET scan, scrubbing my body with surgical soap three different times, and fasting after 7:00pm. I took my last work call at 4:00 Monday afternoon, and Christy and I grabbed a quick meal. As we checked into the hotel in Charleston, we were nervous like before our first date. Neither of us wanted to be the first to break down. We talked, we laughed, we reminisced, and we cried...a lot. While we were always confident that our plan would work, there was still the chance that something could go wrong. The post-surgery recovery plan was also still up in the air. I cannot imagine living my life without my wife by my side and I know she feels the same way.

We arrived at the hospital at 5:30am and were whisked back to the surgery prep area, where Christy and I removed my wedding band (the only time I have removed my ring over the last 21 years was during surgery or scans) and I joked that we would not officially be married during my surgery since I did not have my ring on. I kissed her goodbye for now and told her I would see her in a couple hours. On the way back to the surgical room lying flat on a gurney and seeing all the nurses and doctors both treating me and ready to treat other patients in similar rooms, I was fist bumping anyone I saw, trying to get them hyped up. I am kicking cancer's ass today! I had asked for my favorite Foo Fighters songs to be playing in the surgical room. The next 15 minutes had Times Like These, Everlong, and My Hero blasting as loud as the surgical speakers could handle. I then went to sleep while the surgeons and their teams worked on me. They said it would be 14-18 hours, and it took the full 18.

The cancer type, which we would officially find out in surgery was Eccrine Porocarcinoma (EPC), had spread into my skull and dura layer. *Eccrine Porocarcinoma is a rare type of skin cancer that may occur by chance or may develop from a benign (non-cancerous) skin tumor. Porocarcinoma accounts for **0.005% of all malignant cutaneous tumors (skin cancers)** and arises from eccrine sweat gland tumors. Due to its uncommon onset, EPC can be misdiagnosed as other skin neoplasms, and there is no standardized regimen for treating. The mean age for a patient with EPC is 67.5 years old. About 20% of this type of skin cancer will recur and about 20% will metastasize to regional lymph nodes. There is a mortality rate of 67% in patients with lymph node metastases, ranging in five to 24 months. *https://wjso.biomedcentral.com/articles/10.1186/1477-7819-9-32

Think about these statistics. You have a pretty good chance of hitting the lottery rather than getting this type of cancer. The average age for a patient with this disease is nearly 20 years older than me. Even if we can remove all of the cancer, there is a 20% chance it will come back. The two-year mortality rate is very high (two out of every three patients) and there is no set protocol on how to treat.

WE GOT THIS!!!

I am not going to get into all of the specifics of the surgery but here's the high-level overview: When they started surgery, they felt that the area they needed to remove on my head and skull was a little larger than a fist. However, they did not have clear margins on this first removal, and the second removal which was a round circle around my head about 2cm above my eyebrows, also did not yield clear margins for the cancer.

It turned out, the cancer was much larger and way more invasive than could be seen by the scans prior to surgery. The analogy the doctors used to describe the cancer they removed was that it was similar to how termites eat away at the foundation of a house. My entire skull was removed, a new skull (titanium mesh plate) was inserted and my left lat muscle and associated skin flap were removed from my back and sutured in to my head. The surgery took the full 18 hours and was the largest procedure MUSC had performed. I now have a plate in my head that sets off many alarms, including some electric dog fences (just kidding on this). To determine how big this plate is, put your finger on your right eyebrow and begin to trace your head with your finger over your right ear, straight around to the bump on the back of your head, over your left ear, then back to your left eyebrow.

Also, while the surgeons did a miraculous job, there was another challenge we would have to deal with. I now had a massive wound on my back from the removed lat muscle that was used to cover my head. It was much bigger than anticipated. The nurses and doctors said the wound looked like a shark bite on my back. The back wound measured 27cm long by 22cm wide and was 2cm deep. The doctors said the wound was going to be the biggest challenge we faced in the next couple months. After being around wounds for 15 years, little did I know that this donor site, as well as other wounds, would cause us so many problems from May through December.

Christy was finally able to see me around 1:00 Wednesday morning. While it was a long day for me, it was even longer for her, not to mention our friends and family who were eager to get updates from her on my progress. She cried when she saw me, overcome with emotion both from the fact that I survived, how terrible I looked with the breathing tube still in my throat, and also nervous about the recovery. The ICU staff had to eventually tell her to go back to the hotel (kind term for kicking her out) because she needed to rest up and the emotions were taking a toll on her. The nurses told her that she could not be emotional or cry around me because that would cause anxiousness for me in trying to recover. This journey would be way harder than we were originally told, and that first plan was already going to be a challenge.

We were still not aware of what our new normal would be.

ALWAYS LEARNING LEADER TAKEAWAYS:

Sometimes emotion gets in the way of listening to what others have to say. We want to impart our knowledge on others without fully understanding what they are sharing with us. Other times, we as leaders are not sure the questions to ask, because we don't have enough information, or our emotions, while positive in nature, blur our vision to what is truly important or necessary to know. Both examples are demonstrated within our diagnosis story.

- Ask questions of your team...constantly, but not like an interrogator. Ask them what's going well, what challenges they are facing, what you can do to help, and then something personal, like "How is the family?" or what vacations they have scheduled for the year. Don't offer too much advice on anything they say but truly listen, reflect their words back to them, and set up a follow-up session to discuss all these items in the next 14 days. Listen to understand versus listen to respond.

- Count on things getting messy with any complex project. Even with the best process and best of intentions, things will go sideways. "Control your three-foot world" and focus on tasks and actions that you can have an impact on. I was only able to personally control my attitude and the music selections heading into surgery. While not for everyone, I would rock out to Dave Grohl and his mates heading into one of the darkest days of my life because I could control the music. Everything else was irrelevant. When looking at challenges and opportunities, people tend to stress too much on external factors. Focus on the things you can control, ask for help when needed, and celebrate the small wins that will yield to a giant victory.

VIEW THE PICTURES THAT
CHRONICLE OUR JOURNEY

ALWAYSLEARNINGLEADER.COM/WE-GOT-THIS-PICTURES/

CHAPTER 3

Setting SMART Goals, Ice Chips, & the Dangers of the Stretch Goal Concept
*APRIL 2021 – MAY 2021

After the 18-hour surgery, the first thing I remember is hearing voices. This was about 1:00am on Wednesday. I could not open my eyes due to the anesthesia and pain medication running through my body. I felt sluggish and like I had been run over by a bus. I was trying to talk but the tube in my throat was blocking my speech, and my throat hurt.

I then recognized the most beautiful sound in the world...the voice of my wife Christy, who was outside my ICU room and just seeing me awake for the first time. My arms had been secured to the bed rails and I could not move. After some feeling around with my arms and trying to move things, I was able to free up my right arm. I felt my face, felt this foreign item in my throat and pulled out the tube from my throat. I proceeded to vomit all over myself while lying on the bed with the tube dangling. Removing your own breathing tube while heavily sedated is probably not the smartest thing to do. The nurses and doctors quickly came into the room, shocked that I got my arm out of the bed rail and that I pulled the tube out. They quickly medicated me again and I slept until 7:00am. This was however the first sign to me that I had survived surgery. 25 hours earlier, I was sedated and put to sleep and while we had a good plan in place, I was not sure I would wake up again.

Wednesday morning, I woke up to the voice of Dr. David Zaas while in the ICU. David is a close personal friend and the CEO at MUSC-Charleston. He has helped us with so many things over the years, and he and his family are some of the most special people we have come across. I started talking some gibberish about clocks and what time/day it was. It was just great to hear someone else's voice. Christy came in immediately after with some of the residents and nurses. They wanted to run some additional tests on me as my heart rate was skyrocketing.

Originally, our medical team said we would be in the ICU for five to seven days, then we would transfer to the main floor for another seven days of recovery before discharge. But since the surgical areas on both my head and back were much larger than planned, it would be longer now. Before the surgery, even though we were told that it would probably be 14 days until I was discharged, I told everyone I knew that I would be home in eight days. I had never stayed in a hospital overnight before. I wanted to be in my bed and at home to recover. I was determined to do whatever they needed to discharge me within eight days.

The first couple days in the ICU after surgery were sort of a blur. While my heart rate was still high, it had improved, and we were no longer too concerned with this. I was still groggy from the effects of the surgery. The ICU team told me I needed to walk, eat/drink a little bit, and use the restroom in order to be sent to a general floor. I was not hungry or thirsty at all. This is the first of many times that you will hear my wife's name associated with patience and strength. I was out of it on some pretty heavy medications and pain killers. I just wanted little ice chips (they are called bullet chips and are most commonly found in Chick-Fil-A and Sonic drinks). Luckily, MUSC had this type of ice readily available for their patients. But I only wanted one or a couple chips at a time inserted into my mouth with a plastic spoon. I drove my poor wife crazy with these requests, which would be many times each hour. I would lift my fingers to tell her how many chips I wanted with each spoonful. After a day of feeding me ice chips one or two or three at a time, I think she was ready to dump the bucket of ice on my head.

I made myself get out of bed on Day 3 and walk a wobbly 15 steps to the nursing station and 15 back. I felt like my head was a 20-pound bobblehead and much heavier than I was used to, which made the walk very challenging from a stability perspective. During this initial walk, I realized that I had not seen what my body looked like. I knew I had tubes and wires connected all over me. After completing the brief walk, I forgot to ask for a mirror and went straight to sleep. My wife and nurses had made the decision to cover or remove all mirrors in areas I was going to be in because they were not sure I could handle the sight of my newly formed head and how swollen I was. They wanted to be there in person in case I freaked out about the way I looked.

I made enough progress to transfer to the general floor by the end of that third day. We left the ICU room around 1:00am and came down to the ninth floor. I texted Christy, who was at the hotel, right before I left ICU and told her we were moving on to the next phase. As we were rolling down the hallway, I looked up at the round mirrors attached to the ceiling that show you if someone is coming the other way. You can also see yourself in that same mirror if you are laying on the bed. This was the first time I saw my body with a bunch of machines around me and tubes running multiple directions. While my head now resembled the shape of a rhombus, I was on enough pain pills to think "The hard part is now over, I just need to do whatever it takes to get out of here by Wednesday, my stretch goal." I was wrong on the hard part, as the next eight months would provide us challenge after challenge.

Prior to surgery, I already had a big head and always had a difficult time finding hats that fit well. Now my head was much bigger and so was the challenge. I joked that the lat muscle on top of my head made me one inch taller. We searched XXXL hats on the internet and bought and tried on a bunch of hats and sizes, but none of them came close to fitting. Fortunately, our good friends Jenny and Scott McClendon found a great Carhartt winter hat which actually fit over my new circumference. They were also our first visitors at MUSC, and we greatly appreciated the time spent with them there. It was so good to see some of our best friends after being stuck in a hospital room hours away from our home.

The general floor was where we met Emma and the rest of the nursing and PT staff who cared for us with such extreme diligence and watchfulness at MUSC. Emma is one of the best nurses I have ever witnessed, providing me the good and developmental feedback I needed to hear to get better. Emma was constantly talking to Christy about how she was treating me in the hospital and how Christy would be responsible for many of these things after we went home. We talked about food, what Emma's hobbies were, and other clinical and personal stories. When we were discharged, she walked down with us to the car, helped us get loaded up, and then Emma, Christy and I hugged each other and we cried together. She told us she had never cried when discharging a patient. We were the first. All the nurses who treated us over these eight months were great, but

Emma was special to us and we are so lucky to have met her during this first week of recovery.

I met my aggressive target of being discharged in eight days, and left the hospital on Wednesday, May 5th. But we probably should have waited a little longer. I had set a stretch goal, but the smarter goal for all would have been to stay in the hospital with the trained clinicians for a longer time. When we got home from our 4.5-hour drive from Charleston, we had dinner with our kids, and I was asleep on the recliner by 7:00pm. No beeping noises, nobody coming into my room every two hours for some type of test, and no more hospital food. We did have a VAC (Vacuum Assisted Closure) device for the huge donor site wound on my back, but this was only going to be for a couple of weeks. Or so we thought.

Regarding work, Align was amazing from a support perspective. They told me to return to work when I felt strong and healthy. How fortunate am I to work with a company like this? While my doctors told me I should probably return to work in October at the earliest, I set a stretch goal to return on July 19th, which was less than a week after my last radiation treatment. My wife and doctors said I was crazy to go back that soon. Return to work just days after completing seven weeks of radiation following major surgery? But I was determined to get my mind and body healed to hit this goal no matter what...and I did return to work on this date. But as you will read in the next chapter, this return-to-work date was another stretch goal that I probably should have missed. Instead, I should have hit our medical team's realistic goal of Q4.

I thought I knew what our new normal was, but I should have listened to others and taken their advice. We would continue to search for our new normal.

ALWAYS LEARNING LEADER TAKEAWAYS:

- Goal setting should be done over the course of a week or two spent writing them down, reviewing them, and talking about them with your peers and supervisors. They should be Specific, Measurable, Attainable, Relevant, and Time-bound (SMART). They also should be reviewed each quarter to make sure they are still relevant. One of my personal goals in January was to try to get in better shape (I think everyone has this goal in January), however this goal was no longer relevant in April due to my cancer diagnosis.

- Stretch goals are great but you have to listen to others to make sure they are realistic. I was determined to be discharged in eight days after my original surgery. We hit this stretch goal but it would have been beneficial to have another couple days to get used to my new treatment regimen. And my return to work on July 19th, which was 100% my decision, was too much to handle after radiation took a lot out of us. My doctors and wife told me this was too soon, but I was determined to hit this stretch goal. With stretch goals, the Realistic part is the most important attribute of the SMART acronym. Make sure to identify and handle adjustments and be brave enough to change when necessary.

VIEW THE PICTURES THAT
CHRONICLE OUR JOURNEY

ALWAYSLEARNINGLEADER.COM/WE-GOT-THIS-PICTURES/

CHAPTER 4

Warrior Mentality
*MAY 2021 – AUGUST 2021

May through August of 2021 was definitely a roller coaster.

When we were discharged from MUSC on May 5th, I was prescribed some medications to help with the pain and also prescribed a wound VAC (Vacuum Assisted Closure) for my back wound. This is great technology and something I was very familiar with. The doctor or nurse would put a piece of foam on my back, use a special type of tape to secure the foam, then put a two-inch flat vacuum disc in the middle of the foam. The goal for this was to try and close both the width and depth of the wound as quickly as possible.

Our home health nurse Stella would come three times per week to change out these dressings for us. Stella was born in the Philippines and has over 20 years of nursing experience, most of it in the home health space. She is a sweet conversationalist, and we shared many stories about cooking and parenting through our journey to recovery. I gave her some BBQ products and she would bring us fresh vegetables from her garden. Now most of you who know me understand that the vegetables were for Christy and the kids as I had no vegetables in my diet.

Throughout this cancer journey, I have learned that I have a pretty high tolerance for pain. My good friend Ed Hemphill and I always talked about "Embracing the Suck" when life or work got difficult. I dreaded these VAC changes because of the size of my missing lat wound (27cm long by 22cm wide by 2cm deep). The tape to secure the dressing was outside that perimeter of the wound, which was a very sore and already compromised area. Here is how each dressing change occurred:

1. Stella walks into our bedroom, which now looks like a wound care closet.
2. Stella takes my vitals (blood pressure, oxygen, temperature).
3. I remove my shirt and lay flat on my stomach on the bed. I only wore Columbia PFG button-up shirts from May through August as the material was moisture wicking and the only type of material not to stick to the tape on my back, and the shirt was simple to take on and off.
4. We would turn off the VAC and disconnect the disc on my back from the unit.
5. Stella would carefully start pulling back the tape on the foam dressing and removing the tape from my skin (30-40 minutes).

6. Once the tape was completely off, we would remove the 27x22 cm foam which was now "sucked into the wound" (five minutes).
7. She would cleanse the wound, then start to piece together pieces of the foam to put back into my wound (30 minutes).
8. Tape would be applied to create a VAC seal that we prayed would stay sealed for the full 72 hours so as not to have to repeat the process (10 minutes).

These dressing changes would last up to two hours, and were some of the most uncomfortable times I have experienced. It was common that I had pain levels of eight out of 10 or higher with the tape being removed from already compromised places on the back. Stella was great at helping with this difficult process, and always did as much as she could to gently take the tape off, but it always felt like ripping to me.

The VAC definitely did help with reducing the size and depth of the wound, but I was a challenge. The contours of my back and the location made it very difficult to maintain a seal for more than 36 hours. A typical week found us going through the VAC changes four times instead of three. Many times, the nurses would have to try two or three different changes at one time to re-do the dressing change and obtain that seal we needed. When I would lay down for the treatment, knowing how it was going to hurt, I would turn the TV on, and mutter the two quotes that got me through all the tough times:

"Feed the Courage Wolf" and "I can do all things through Christ who gives me strength". The second quote was shared by our good friend Marcus Gleaton, who also is beating cancer.

I now had a sidekick everywhere I went...a nine-pound machine that was sucking out the moisture, mostly red/pink in color, from underneath the VAC foam dressing through the tubes connected to my back. These fluids would rest in a canister on the device which hung over my shoulder until full and then we would exchange canisters to start the process over again. I likened having this VAC "accessory" to a fanny pack, which my hip teenage daughter said was coming back in style. I mean they sell fanny packs at Lululemon so they must be in style, right?

We started radiation treatment at UNC Hospital in Chapel Hill on May 24th. Typically, radiation is set for a specific small area to target the cancer cells. My situation was going to be different. Because they removed such a large area on my head, coupled with the fact that our surgeons were not able to remove the part of the tumor near the sagittal sinus vein in my head, my whole head would have to be treated with radiation and we needed to get started as soon as possible. Side effects could include dizziness, sleep difficulties, nausea, headaches, radiation burn, potential loss of taste, delayed wound healing, possible seizures or strokes, and loss of appetite. These side effects could impact me in the current state or at any time without warning in the coming years.

The week before radiation treatments began, I was brought into UNC-Chapel Hill and fitted for a mask that would have me bolted to the flat bed of the radiation machine. This mask would not let my head move a millimeter for 25 minutes per day for seven weeks, Monday through Friday. The mask was somewhat intimidating to look at (think of Hannibal Lecter in shape and style), it was awkward to get fitted for, and even more interesting to have me bolted securely to each day.

For each radiation treatment, Christy would drive me the 45 minutes to the hospital, as I still could not drive with the multiple prescriptions I was taking. I would enter the radiation oncology office, scan my card, and wait for the nurses to come get me and bring me back to a room with a big machine and a lot of monitors. The room was very dark and somber with very thick gray cement walls. Things did seem to get better when we started cranking Foo Fighters songs. The nurse's energy picked up as did mine. After treatment, we would drive the 45 minutes home.

The unique challenge I had to manage through radiation was that I had this huge wound on my back with the VAC device. I also did not have a left lat muscle to move my left arm too well. The nurses would gingerly move me to the flat board I had to lay on through each treatment, with my VAC device located between my feet on the board. I then had to shuffle left, right, up, or down to make sure I was positioned appropriately on the board. Next, each arm had to hold a handle to stretch toward my feet for the entire treatment, as my shoulders needed to be pulled down away from my head. Finally, the techs put the custom mask on my head and secured me with four bolts to the board. This occurred every weekday for seven weeks. We were positive that Dr. Chera and his team had a great plan and these seven weeks sort of flew by. We experienced a lot of pain and discomfort, much of which my doctors and nursing staff were impressed that I could handle. I was called a warrior by these therapists helping me to improve each day. To me, a warrior is a person who will succeed in any ethical way possible, no matter the obstacle. I was going to live up to that descriptor and was honored to be considered in this way.

I also had to deal with the fact that I would spend these seven weeks surrounded by Carolina blue for an hour per day. Chapel Hill is a beautiful college town, with its campus and hospital dominated by this light blue color. After attending NC State University 30 miles to the east in Raleigh, I had learned to detest this shade of blue as well as most things UNC-related. This "loathing" of UNC-Chapel Hill and the Carolina blue color had also been adopted by my son. When we moved back to the Raleigh area in 2013, we purchased a great home in Wake Forest. The room that would be Connor's was painted Carolina blue. He told us there was no way he would ever sleep in that room. Christy and I pointed out that we could paint the room any color he wanted, but he still argued that he would not sleep in that room, knowing that the Carolina blue color would be underneath whatever color he decided on. Christy and I got quite a kick out of his stance, and I was actually proud of him for it, but he finally relented, we repainted the room, and everything turned out fine with our new home.

But I still had to endure the Carolina blue for my daily MRI treatments. One of my best friends, Doug Scott, had listened to my concerns about having this temporary exposure to Carolina blue in my life. An All-American decathlete at NC State in the early 90's, he too had a dislike for the color. So, he sent me something that would help ease my pain. I received a box from Doug the day before my first radiation treatment, containing a pair of sunglasses with red lenses. While wearing them, I would see everything in NC State red. It was the perfect gift for us as we prepared for seven weeks of Carolina blue!!!

I mentioned some of the potential side effects of radiation of my head. I only experienced two during treatment, and one of them was only temporary, but both were difficult, and one would have long-term effects on my healing process. The temporary side effect was radiation burn on my head. Imagine going to the beach on a hot summer day and getting sunburned on your forehead. The next day, you do it again, having the sun's rays burn your head again in the same place. You are also limited to the lotions you can put on in between days in the sun to help reduce the pain. I was sunburned on my forehead from the radiation for the last six weeks of treatment. We tried multiple UNC-approved treatments for the burn, but none of them worked for me. Christy spent hours researching the best lotions or products for radiation burn and we tried a number of them, but nothing worked. My forehead was a dark shade of maroon and was extremely uncomfortable. However, this was temporary and something we could get through.

The long-term complication was that the radiation to my head had opened up my surgery incision site. This wound, stretching around my head from the front to the back was now split open, with dead tissue inside. Delayed wound healing because of radiation is very common. We could not treat these new head wounds until after radiation was completed.

We had an extra day off from radiation on the long July 4th weekend, and took advantage of it for a change of scenery. We love going to the beach, and we were going to reunite with some friends from Texas. The Simmons family is one of the sweetest we know, and we have taken many vacations and cruises with them in our 15 years of friendship. We had originally planned to be at the beach for 10 days, but the radiation schedule of daily treatments had us alter that to only three. In addition, this beach trip had me confined to a recliner in the living room. I could not go to the beach, and I had to limit my interactions with other people due to chance of infection. I still loved being there with our great friends, saw some excellent fireworks from our home, and enjoyed my break from the radiation board.

Before we knew it, July 13th was upon us. That was the last day of radiation. We could not wait to bang the gong, symbolic of completing radiation at UNC Hospital. It was a great day for our family as I slowly beat the mallet into the cymbal, to a crescendo of noise and one final bang on the gong. Getting those 2.5 hours a day back was life-changing. Christy and I look back and we are still amazed with how we managed our time. Now we had to wait until October to see if the combination of surgery and radiation worked. While this seemed like a long time to wait for the results, we understood this was standard protocol.

Not heeding the advice of my wife and doctors, I returned to work on July 19th, three months ahead of schedule. Align had been so supportive of me and I felt it was my obligation to return the gesture in getting back to my job. I tried to get back to normal, still with this open gap around my head. I started going out to dinners with my family, driving (I was off my pain pills), and getting stuff ready for Connor to go off to college in mid-August.

The MUSC surgical team and I were scheduled to meet the first week of August to discuss how to treat the wounds on my head and back. But before that could happen, on August 1st we were delivered a knockout blow that our doctors and nurses said should have killed me…and was worse than anything we had been through the last four months.

ALWAYS LEARNING LEADER TAKEAWAYS:

I have stated many times that I am never the smartest person in the room. As a leader, I would surround myself with people who were honest, dependable, accountable and offered a different perspective than I did. I listened and learned, which led me to make better and more informed decisions. However, I would rarely be out-worked or out-hustled in any position and I loved taking on roles, projects, or jobs that other people did not want or did not succeed in before me. I felt my attitude and effort were twice as important as the God-given talent I possessed.

Whenever I hired a new team member, I treated this new hire with tremendous appreciation. They were committing their career and professional happiness/ development to our organization and to me, and I would do my best not to let them down. After four to six months in their new role, I would ask the new hire if the position was exactly like what we talked about during the interview process. A lot of times, they said it was better than what we had discussed. This was the desired outcome. If they felt the position was different, I knew I had to reset how I positioned any new role with future candidates.

I enjoy the grind and the process, and building legacies for the professional work we accomplish as a team. Regarding our current health situation, we could not have beaten cancer without sheer grit and determination from everyone around me. We knew what the end result was going to be when we originally heard the news. One of my dear friends, Laura Ackerman, shared "Cancer picked the wrong bald man" and she was right.

- We all have that warrior mentality in us for something. It could be fighting for a cause that means a lot to us or to fight and protect a family member. Typically, this warrior mentality comes alive when a person is passionate about the task at hand. This passion permeates into their daily activities and they will fight to the end until they reach their final destination, whether it is planning a meeting at work, fighting for more diversity and equality for others, or if they are enduring the pain to get all the cancer out of their body. The takeaway is hire and develop people in positions that they enjoy and are good at. It honestly is that simple.

- Don't Go Solo – (credit to MZ for this concept). Leading others is something you should not do alone. I believe the most important job any leader has is hiring the right people. When a leader makes a bad personnel decision, they will spend more time working with the C player versus their A players. Leaders also need to share successes and failures with others. Show me a leader who says they have never made a bad hire, and I will tell you about a unicorn I saw running on I-40 in

North Carolina last week. Spend time on interviewing skills, listening skills, and trying to hire the best team possible. Also, never interview alone. It is always great to have another team member or peer with you, whether that's in person or in a Zoom room, to consider the candidate from a different lens.

VIEW THE PICTURES THAT
CHRONICLE OUR JOURNEY

ALWAYSLEARNINGLEADER.COM/WE-GOT-THIS-PICTURES/

CHAPTER 5

The Knockout Punch
*AUGUST 2021

Sunday, August 1st was a beautiful hot summer day in Wake Forest, NC. The sun was shining and we had just spent two days with Christy's brother Matthew, his wife Jessie, and their three-year-old son Jackson. We had not seen them in person for 18 months due to Covid and it was great to reconnect. They left around 10:00am for their four-hour drive back to Asheville. As I had returned to work, I took an hour to review my upcoming week for follow-up appointments. I had a busy week ahead as I was just starting to get back to the job I loved doing. I was looking forward to a lunch meeting on Monday with two of my favorite people in the industry, Dr. Jason Gladwell and Jennifer Pinder, who I had known for years. Dr. Gladwell was one of the people who confirmed to me how great a company Align was and that I had to work for them. Dr. Gladwell, Jennifer and their team have the most impressive marketing program I have seen in the medical industry, and Align was looking to partner with them on some upcoming education. They are also great people and friends. I knew seeing them would kick off a great week.

I proceeded to cook lunch for our family, and then retreated to my La-Z-Boy recliner, where I had slept the majority of the last three months due to the VAC on my back. I was not comfortable sleeping flat in our bed with the disc and foam from the VAC, and the recliner that Christy and the kids bought for me the day before I left for surgery was a game changer for me. I fell asleep for a nap around 1:30 in the afternoon.

All in all, I had felt pretty good during the last two weeks of July. We had finally moved away from the VAC on my back, changing to moist dressings two times per day. It was still a large site but we were planning to eventually do a skin graft for this. The incision site on my head continued to be split open between the flap on top of my head and my forehead. Approximately half of this incision site was open but covered with necrotic (dead) tissue. Now that radiation was complete, we could start treating the wounds on my head. We had an appointment later that week at MUSC to set up a game plan for next steps.

I woke up after about an hour and immediately felt different. I was sweating, and felt like the wind was knocked out of me when I stood up. There was also a foul smell that I was all too familiar with, wound infection. I texted Christy, who was on the Peloton upstairs, that I was feeling terrible. She came straight down the steps, took one look at me, and took my temperature. The digital readout showed 103.6 degrees. She took it again and it was 103.7 degrees. I texted my good friend Dot Weir, who had offered us some great advice and support for our wounds and is one of the most genuine and caring people I know. Dot said for me to get to the closest emergency room immediately. By then I had gone from sweating to freezing. I walked outside on a sunny August day with temperatures in the high 90's, but I needed a sweatshirt for the chills I was feeling.

We decided to go to UNC Hospital in Chapel Hill, as we had completed radiation there and they would have my information in their system. Our main doctors were at MUSC in Charleston, 4.5 hours away, which was too far to drive in my current condition. We felt fortunate that the doctors at UNC and MUSC were communicating from the April surgery to present day to determine what was best for me.

We drove the 45 minutes to UNC Hospital, were admitted to the ER and hooked up to an IV in each arm. They started me on fluids and we saw a doctor who looked at me with amazement. She had never heard of Porocarcinoma, and had never seen a patient like me, with a huge back wound and a head shaped like a rhombus that was half good tissue and half dead tissue around the incision site. She could immediately smell the infection, so they cultured several parts of the wound to determine just what the infection was. I also now had an area on the side of my head that was slowly collecting fluid. Before they started me on fluids and antibiotics, the staff wanted me to go through some scans on my head and body. We had three different scans that night, the last one around 1:00am. We were still in the ER on the gurney bed, which was so uncomfortable. Life had definitely changed direction from how I felt about 12 hours earlier.

We wound up remaining in the ER for 30 hours after admission. With Covid and nursing shortages, the hospital was unable to find a bed for me. While extremely uncomfortable, I understood what they were going through. The nurses who were there were doing their best to get me transferred, but sometimes things get bottlenecked, especially in the summer of 2021.

Based on the test results, two different types of infections were flowing through my body. I was on multiple antibiotics and would have a surgical procedure bedside to drain the pocket of fluid on the side of my head. This took place on Tuesday, two days after admission into the emergency room.

We also had to do a lumbar puncture, sometimes referred to as a spinal tap, to make sure that my cerebral spinal fluid was not leaking. I know women deal with this procedure a lot during childbirth, but, in my opinion, women are stronger than men when it comes to these types of things. I was dreading this procedure that would have two doctors slowly plunge a needle into the lower part of my back and drain enough fluid out to test. They said depending on the speed of the flow drip (some patients are free flowing and some drip at a snail's pace), the procedure could last anywhere from 15-45 minutes. I think you can guess which group I was in.

I was using the TV to time events. I would watch 30-minute sitcoms to break up my days into chunks. About 30 minutes after the needle was inserted, I asked the doctors how it was going. I had to cough as I had some fluid in my throat from lying on my side during the procedure, and asked them if I could do that. They said no, I could not cough or sneeze due to the huge needle stuck in my back. And no surprise, they told me I was probably the slowest spinal tap they had ever done and we were only about halfway to acquiring the right amount of fluid to test. It took about 50 minutes for the entire procedure to be complete. As soon as it was over, I think I coughed and sneezed at the same time! Luckily, these cerebral spinal tests were negative and we moved on to try to handle the other infections and problems in my body.

For the next five days, I was pumped with many antibiotics, each one equipped to help me fight off the infections and get me feeling well enough so my body could handle the five-hour ambulance ride from UNC Hospital in Chapel Hill, NC to MUSC in Charleston, SC. Another problem was now occurring that was unique to me. I am a tough patient to draw blood from or to insert an IV into. I am not an infectious disease doctor, but I believe the number of fluids and the type of the fluids they were administering through the IVs were wreaking havoc on my veins. It seems like we would put an IV in one arm, and would have to insert another one into my other arm within 48 hours to help assist with administration of the antibiotics.

Word of my difficult veins whispered through the nursing staff on the seventh floor, and all the nurses were nervous about inserting an IV into my arm, where they might fail and have to try again. They now had to call in their special IV team to insert IVs into my arms using ultrasound technology. It was a very good decision...it worked well, and this protocol followed me to MUSC. The team at UNC was wonderful, and I was loaded into the ambulance for the drive to MUSC on August 10th, nine days after being admitted to the emergency room at UNC.

After the longest five-hour drive of my life, spent lying on a gurney and two-inch rubber mattress, facing backwards, in pain from the wound on my back and answering the many questions from my EMT tech who was trying to figure out how my health had deteriorated, I was admitted to MUSC. We had been in constant communication with the MUSC team while in the hospital at UNC and now had a new surgery scheduled for August 12th.

We were hoping that just one four-hour operation would be able to close the gaps in my head caused by the radiation and eliminate the infection. After clearing out the dead tissue in the wound bed around my head and temporarily shifting the flap to clean out areas of concern underneath the flap, the plastic surgeons would have to pull my forehead up and reattach the skin flap. These were some pretty sizable gaps they had to try to close. The combination of stitches and staples used had my head looking like railroad tracks. I woke up from surgery, and as the anesthesia subsided, I noticed two new pain points I had not had before I went to sleep for surgery. One was how bad my forehead felt due to the stretching upwards. Secondly, I felt something very different in my right ankle. Even with the talented IV nurses looking for veins in my arms, we were still having some challenges due to the antibiotics running through the IV tubing. During surgery, our surgeons had decided that the healthiest vein where an IV could be inserted was above my right ankle bone. I am glad I was knocked out for that procedure.

After this surgery, I was extremely sore. My head and ankle throbbed in pain, my back was hurting as the wound had stalled healing, and my energy level was down to about one out of 10. And we now had a new challenge at home. Connor would start his freshman year of college in two weeks, and athletes had to report to campus in just a few days. Christy would have to drive 4.5 hours home and help her first-born pack up for college in one day. This is a very emotional experience for most moms, and given our situation, was even more so. But she did it. That Sunday, Christy and Kelcie drove the two hours from Wake Forest, NC to Farmville, VA, helped Connor move into his dorm room (on the third floor of one of the oldest dorms in the country, with no elevator), and then drove home. Christy would then drive back to Charleston, SC on Monday to resume taking care of me. Have you learned yet how incredible my wife is with managing our schedules???

My sister Suzanne had come to Charleston to look after me for the two days that Christy was not there, buy me ice cream, and tell me about some better pain reducing options for what I was dealing with. This is just another example of everyone chipping in to help us. This is a new concept for our family as we were typically the givers of support when asked, and have rarely been on the receiving end because we are blessed beyond measure. I cannot remember the last time I was sick prior to cancer, and while we have definitely asked for last-minute help in the past for our dogs to be let out or for our mail to be picked up, it was not common. The support we were receiving was AMAZING. Dinners were provided almost every night for four months. Carpools were set up for school and soccer. Now that Connor was off to college, we could not leave my precious angel Kelcie at home by herself. Sleepovers and help with school were left to our dear friends in Wake Forest. To everyone who cooked or provided meals and support to us (and the list is very long), Thank You!

At first, we were uncomfortable, and almost embarrassed, receiving all this help. We had never needed much help in the past, and now we could not function without it. There were others in our community who needed help more than us. But I soon learned that these acts of kindness were not about us and our feelings. The people who supported us got such a high from helping us, that it made them feel good, similar to how Christy and I felt when we did a good deed for others.

Christy arrived in Charleston around noon on Monday. Some additional scans conducted over the weekend would show that surgeons had to go back in and clean out the areas in my head some more. I would undergo another four-hour surgery Tuesday, August 17th. It was scheduled for 11:00am but it started late, and I didn't return to my room until around 5:00. I was exhausted again, my forehead still hurt and the IV was still in my ankle. This surgery also re-introduced an old friend to us, the Wound VAC. Instead of being on my large back wound, a smaller version of the VAC was now on the back of my head. To paint a picture of what this looked like, think back to the first Matrix movie where Neo had the plug in the back of his head on the ship. It was even more uncomfortable than the VAC I had on my back in May and June. We also had issues with the seal on this wound, and the tape removal process was the same painful experience we had previously dealt with.

I had been in either UNC Hospital or MUSC Hospital for 17 straight days. During this time, I had IVs in eight different sites on my arms and one on my ankle. IV fluids were constantly flowing through me. I had blood drawn by the phlebotomists before 6:00 every morning. I jokingly referred to them as the vampires that would sneak into my room just as I had fallen into a deep REM phase of sleep, silently walk up beside me, stick my hands to get the blood sample they needed from me, and sneak out. They were great, but I was looking forward to not having to be stuck any more once home.

We were discharged on August 18th with a follow-up visit scheduled back with the surgery team seven days later, the date of our 21st wedding anniversary. MUSC installed a PICC line in my right arm for Christy to administer one of the antibiotics I would be on for the next 21 days. I also had a host of other medications I was taking orally to try to officially defeat this infection once and for all.

Christy and I saw our medical team in person at MUSC the next week. I was walking around a little bit but still in pain as they assessed my progress, which to them was very positive. I, on the other hand, felt defeated and that we had taken a bunch of steps backward. I used the analogy that I was at the 13-mile mark of a 26-mile marathon, and had just received a penalty that I had to go back and run miles 10-13 again. I asked Dr. Day, who was the main coordinator of my treatment, what he thought. His answer was "You should not be standing here today. That infection should have killed you. You have an amazing wife and great support team behind you. You have dealt with obstacles and hurdles we could not have accounted for, and you have done it with a smile on your face. You are a warrior and it is a miracle you are still alive."

We were knocked down but we were not going to be knocked out!!!

ALWAYS LEARNING LEADER TAKEAWAYS:

- **Events + Reaction = Outcome:** August 1st through 18th were the longest 18 days of our cancer journey. I was sick in multiple places with wounds on my back and head to heal, infections flowing through my body, and having to rebuild my stamina. The effects from radiation will continue to impact my body years after our last treatment, and I began to experience tremors in my hands and massive headaches that would randomly impact me. **Events** would hit us, our surgical and support team would **react** to these events, and make a plan for a positive **outcome**. This equation is something I have used for years both personally and with our family as we deal with situations, whether they are positive, developmental, or challenging. For me, having a negative **reaction** to **events** that were outside of my control was not helpful. I also chose to only see or talk to the people who could share that same mindset. Think about the **events** in your life. Take a moment to reflect on your best **reactions** (it does not have to be an immediate response) to result in a positive **outcome**.

- In March and April, I would have people ask me if I was mad that I got cancer. That thought never crossed our mind as that was an **event** that was now past us, and one that I had no control over. Having a negative **reaction** to an **event** you don't control or was in the past typically does not yield anything other than negative **outcomes**. A leader can still conduct an After-Action Review of a controlled negative outcome to insure it does not happen again. Never once have we asked "Why us?" I trusted this small group of friends as the core group of people I would talk to on the phone or on Facetime when the shit was hitting the fan. Cancer was the hand we were dealt. The only outcome we focused on was healing and remission, and doing it with a smile on my face and saying "Thank you."

VIEW THE PICTURES THAT
CHRONICLE OUR JOURNEY

ALWAYSLEARNINGLEADER.COM/WE-GOT-THIS-PICTURES/

CHAPTER 6

The Team, Missed Experiences, & October 11ᵗʰ

*AUGUST 2021 – OCTOBER 2021

"I am a member of a team, and I rely on the team, I defer to it and sacrifice for it, because the team, not the individual, is the ultimate champion."
-Mia Hamm

How many teams are you a part of? I heard this question asked during a recent podcast Christy and I were listening to while driving to Charleston. We had stopped listening to music and started listening to books on tape and podcasts, which seems to make the drive a lot shorter in our minds. We listen to a variety of topics, from a DiSC podcast, to Matthew McConaughey's Green Lights to Kevin Hart making us laugh for three hours.

The question was posed around the recognition perspective, based on having even the slightest of impact on others. I would say I am on five teams within Christy's family and mine, 10 teams with my friends' groups from across the country, three teams with my position on the NCFC board of directors, and no less than 25 teams for work. I lead some of these teams, and I am an active participant in the rest. That is a total of 43 teams I figured I was a part of before surgery. Now add an additional 15 teams I am on with treating my cancer (surgical team, PT team, home health team, radiation team, infection disease team, etc.), and I know I probably missed some while reviewing this.

Teamwork has always been important to me. As a High I on the DiSC profile for most of my life, I love to work with others toward a common objective. There were times when I was not a productive member of a team, but I am confident that I have been a positive leader/influencer on most teams I have been selected to lead or participate in.

There are two things I think are critical to have on a successful team, besides the standard Purpose and Process aspects that we try to aspire to for all of our interactions.

- All team members' views are important and should be taken into account before a decision is made. The leader is ultimately the one who has to make the final decision as they should be the one accountable, but a leader who does not listen more than they talk during meetings is going to struggle with their team's output and vision for the project.

- Recognition of the team has to be immediate (depending on the situation, it should be done within 24 hours), often, and specific. Each leader should set aside 15 minutes per day to send out some kind of recognition to three to five people on their team or peer members. It could also be to a friend you have not seen in a while, thanking them for their friendship. If you can't find three to five people a day, you are not looking hard enough at the teams you are on. Specific feedback is a skill you will develop the more you provide it to others. When we used to have our reps and managers conduct live roleplays in training, we would have the class provide the first five observations about what they just saw. The typical response was "They did good". This vague reply offered no help to the recipient. We then shifted gears that would make the observers provide a better review of the roleplay performance. Called the 2+1 rule, each viewer's response had to include two positive and one developmental observation. After the feedback was given to the recipient, the recipient could only say "Thank you," and we would continue the loop. Part of this feedback exercise was also built around the ability to receive feedback without getting defensive.

This feedback modification turned around how we viewed these sessions, while still in a developmental and safe space. Observers were forced to pay closer attention to the roleplay and the feedback loop was received extremely well. I can tell you there was only one time in five years and countless classes that a peer observer was cruel and inappropriately provided particularly negative feedback to the person in the roleplay chair, essentially throwing that participant "under the bus". That peer observer was no longer with the company 14 days later.

My wife has always been the leader of our household. When people would ask me on a Friday afternoon about my weekend plans, my reply typically was "Whatever my wife tells me to do". With my diagnosis, she now became the unquestioned leader of everything "Jimmy Cancer" related including:

- Updates on Jimmy's health by text message or phone calls.
- Coordination of wound care, PT and radiation appointments.
- Administering of medications, which I still take three times per day.
- Wound dressing changes (one to two times per day at 30-60 minutes per dressing change).
- Ordering of new supplies for wound treatments.

- Slowing me down when I was pushing too hard to get back to normal.

She managed all of this while sometimes being 4.5 hours away, being a mother to two teenagers, running a successful real estate business, and riding the Peloton five days a week. Through her leadership, we established text chat groups, segmented by immediate family, extended family, work, friend groups in NC and TX, Jimmy's fraternity brothers and a few others, each with a team leader. This process worked great, and hopefully was made personal by having team leaders share messages with others. We also explained the process to our friends so they would realize we were trying to be resourceful with the time that was flying by. Everyone understood we could not talk personally to every friend or family member. I think this made us all more efficient, kept everyone informed, and was specific to what we were going through.

I mentioned the multiple teams we were on within our care community. Being a nurse today is an insanely difficult job, no matter if you are in long-term care, home health, or a hospital setting. Nursing is typically thankless as nurses are only treating people who are sick or recovering from sickness and not in the best of moods. In my years of working with clinicians to improve clinical outcomes, I knew the nurses were the backbone to getting patients better. Being the patient gave me a whole new appreciation for these warriors in scrubs. More than 95% of my total time of treatment, surgery and recovery in hospitals was spent with the nursing staff. Less than five percent was spent with doctors.

Christy and I started making sure we said "Thank you" after every nurse or nursing assistant interaction. We always shared that while we were only on the nurse's floor for a temporary stay, we were a member of the nurse's team and we would only get better together during this short time. We would find out the hospital's recognition program and submit multiple names and specific reasons for why we filled out the form or wrote a letter. We laughed with them, and when they had to hurt me to get me better, I tried to handle it with a smile. An example: I had to get a shot in my stomach two times per day after the April surgery to prevent blood clots as I was pretty much bed-bound for the eight days I was there. On day three, there was significant bruising, with the outline of what looked like a pumpkin. I then said, "Let's try to make a bruise pumpkin with each shot." Obviously, all shots were administered properly, but this gave me the chance to a take a "poke" at something which was miserable and make it fun.

Once we were discharged from MUSC on August 18th, our focus was on rest and building back up my energy levels. I had to get the VAC on the back of my head changed three times per week, and Christy was administering my antibiotics through the PICC line inserted into my arm. Since she had to be the one to plunge four different vials into my arm every couple hours for three weeks, she could not go see Connor at college in Virginia, or visit her family in Asheville. Due to the risk of the infection coming back, I was pretty much quarantined to our home until October 1st. I was also taking multiple medications which did not allow me to drive. One day per week, I would have a friend pick me up and we would just take a drive for a few hours to get me out of the house, as I was going stir-crazy.

Cancer caused me to miss many events, including moving my son into college, attending any of Kelcie's or Connor's soccer games for months, and most importantly, taking my wife out to a nice dinner on our anniversary. Our 21st anniversary was the first one where that didn't happen. Plus, many routine things were not allowed, such as lifting items weighing more than 10 pounds. It was tough for me to cook, carry our laundry up the stairs, or hold the leashes as we walked our 80-pound and 60-pound dogs. Christy's role as my wife was now redefined as a caregiver. As much as I tried to lift a basket, or clean up pans after dinner, she sternly but politely told me to sit down and relax. She is an unbelievable woman.

I always enjoy a glass of wine, beer, or a favorite bourbon a few times a week. We asked our infectious disease doctor if I could enjoy an adult beverage or two while taking these multiple antibiotics. He immediately said "Absolutely not," and informed us that alcohol of any kind, even mouthwash, would cause me to get violently sick. Sometimes doctors or nurses are cautious and overstate the negative side effects tied in with medications. But that wasn't the case here. A quick Google search about mixing these medications with alcohol confirmed the negative effects our doctor warned us about. No alcohol until 2022.

While I was missing our kids' games (and the occasional drink), I tried to fill that time with timelining our journey. There are many tears and thoughts that go through your mind with an After-Action review of this nature. It was difficult and cathartic. I realized the extent of what we had been through, and that Christy and I should take pride in how we handled cancer. But I greatly missed my job and working with the Align education team and our faculty.

Physical therapy started for me September 14th. Our therapist Ellen would come to our home three times per week to help me try to rebuild my lat muscle. Ellen is a no-nonsense physical therapist who used to work for the Baltimore Orioles. In her 50's, she is in fantastic physical shape. She works out seven days a week, something many people younger than her can't do. Ellen also has a hobby of training dogs, and I was often embarrassed by the behavior of our dogs when she would ring our doorbell.

Our sessions were one hour, and I think she had every minute planned out. I loved this type of regimented plan. She is my type of clinician. We talked about purpose and process. There was still a stalled wound around 15cm by 10cm on my back where my lat muscle once was, and I had not really moved my left arm or shoulder much since April. We needed to avoid "frozen shoulder" which would possibly mean another surgery or more extensive PT. I was able to dress myself using just my right arm, but any activities requiring my left arm had been non-existent for six months as I moved all physical responsibilities to my right arm. Ellen and I started with some basic range of motion exercises and stretches to improve my left shoulder. I had homework for the days we were not together, which included a detailed plan of how many stretches and how many sets to complete.

Here is another example of how a stretch goal or trying to accomplish something too quickly can hurt you. On my off days, if Ellen said to do 10 stretches per set and three sets per day, I would double it. My daughter would laugh at me, saying that every time she saw me in the house, I was stretching on the countertops, or touching the moldings above the door, which were the stretches Ellen was having me do. I was convinced I would wake up the muscles around the lat muscle to get them more flexible. More importantly, I was going to prove to Ellen that I could handle anything she threw my way and I was going to be tougher than she was.

This was a mistake. With me overdoing it, my shoulder actually starting hurting more and I threw my lower back out. I now needed help getting up from the La-Z-Boy, and walked around the house like a 90-year-old man for three days until the next time I saw Ellen. When she came for her next visit, I slowly walked to the door to let her in, and she quickly asked me what I had done. She scolded me for not following her plan, I agreed, and then we turned to next steps on how to get better.

We also found out that some of the stretches, while good for the muscles in my back, were causing recently healed areas of the wound on my back to stretch and reopen. Nothing critical but we quickly moved the therapy sessions to only tasks that would not cause further harm to my back wound.

It was soon October 11th, the day I would have scans performed to tell us the results of the surgery plus radiation plan, covering April 27th through July 13th. We were confident in the plan we chose, and were cautiously optimistic as we arrived at UNC at 7:30am. I was taken back to the imaging center. They placed an IV in my arm, and I was sent to the MRI room first. After lying on the board for 45 minutes, I was quickly transferred to another room for the CT scan, which took another 10 minutes on the board. Christy and I would know the results sometime that day.

We told our friends and family that we would not know the results from these scans until later that week, to give us time to digest the news before we updated everyone, whether the news was positive or negative. Our clinicians had told us that when you get the news from a scan, pray and hope for the best but prepare for the worst. For my situation, I still also had to deal with three open wounds on my head and one on my back, with surgery scheduled for the back wound October 19th. Whatever the news would be from the MRI, we would still have some major hurdles to overcome with healing the wounds.

Positive news from the MRI could include:
- The tumor was significantly smaller (50% or greater reduction in size). This scenario had the highest probability.
- The cancer was in complete remission. This was the least probable outcome.

Negative news could include:
- The tumor had grown or is the same size.
- The cancer had spread to other areas of our body.
  - Both of these scenarios were still very possible due to our cancer type.

Christy and I drove most of the way home from Chapel Hill holding hands and thinking through the journey of the last six months. What we had been through was harder than we could have ever imagined, with unforeseen challenges hitting us multiple times in this path to complete healing. With Porocarcinoma, there is not an established protocol for treatment or healing. It challenged our surgeons and doctors to be agile with how we treated both the cancer and the wounds associated with it. As we looked back, we both felt proud of the resiliency we had displayed, and extremely humbled by the support from our friends and our caregivers. Being humbled can many times be associated with a negative event. While we were humbled by the power and ferocity of how cancer took over my body and invaded my skull, we felt that the humbleness from the acts of kindness shown to us far exceeded any of our expectations.

Connor was home for Fall Break and we were going to have lunch with him before he headed back to Virginia for a late-afternoon practice. He was taking me to pick up a prescription, then we would come home and pick up Christy. As we were heading home, my cell phone rang at 11:42am. It was Dr. Chera, who was our Radiation Oncologist at UNC. He had just taken a look at our MRI, and it showed our cancer was in complete remission!!! I asked him to repeat what he had just said on speaker phone and he repeated those same words. Connor and I fist bumped and he said "I told you that We Got This". I told Connor to hurry home as this was news I had to tell Christy in person. We made it home in record time.

When I told my lovely wife the update, we laughed, cried, and embraced for what felt like an hour, but was actually only a couple minutes. We had fought together, as a team, and she was my leader. I have always admired her, but her leading our entire team to get to this remission outcome was one of the most incredible and generous displays I have seen or heard of. She had created an environment and a team culture that allowed me to heal, while also managing the process of scheduling everything with my care and notifying others. While the ultimate day of celebration will eventually be when I wake up in no pain and my body is completely closed of all open wounds, we celebrated this major victory which gave us renewed hope.

In talking with Dr. Chera at UNC, he was pretty shocked about the results, obviously in a very good way. Even though we had confidence in the plan we created, to see and experience the plan work is something pretty special. We shared this remission news with the MUSC team. They were pleasantly surprised as well. Family and friends were next. It was a great couple days.

Our New Normal was taking shape.

ALWAYS LEARNING LEADER TAKEAWAYS:

Below are two quotes from one of my favorite people (Leigh S.) on the culture we tried to instill for teams I led. I met Leigh very early in her sales career, and immediately knew she was going to be something special to our company. We worked together for many years and she has not disappointed on any project we worked on. Even though we work for different companies now, we still talk once a month. She recently shared with me a couple things she remembered about our time in the trenches, especially around creating a positive work environment, earning trust and delivering recognition. I have learned as much from her over the years as she has learned from me.

- **Elevate and Recognize Your People** - "When I worked for you, we worked a lot. There were no 40-hour work weeks. Sometimes we'd be in class all day and then study hall all night. It was round-the-clock when we had a class and yet, we didn't feel the burden. We felt like part of the mission; valued, trusted and elevated to get a glimpse into what could be and potentially impact that. You found ways to make us feel special...a dinner at your home, chair massages in the middle of Train-The-Trainer, RST iPods for Carmen and me...those little things went a long way."
- **Is this your best work?** - "I remember completing an assignment for you and when I

sent it in, I asked you what you thought and you said, "Is this your best work?" Of course, that threw me for a loop, and I went back and reread it and brushed it up some more. After re-sending to you, you asked again if this was my best work, and I confidently responded "Yes." You replied, "Because if it's your best work, I don't need to read it". What that taught me was you believed in my work and trusted me to deliver a solid product, whatever it was. It tapped into my internal drivers to be exceptional without you having to give me one word of feedback. So transformational."

VIEW THE PICTURES THAT
CHRONICLE OUR JOURNEY

ALWAYSLEARNINGLEADER.COM/WE-GOT-THIS-PICTURES/

CHAPTER 7

Perspective & Priorities
*OCTOBER 2021

Back in April 2021, three weeks after originally learning about my cancer diagnosis, I was scheduled for a second MRI at UNC-Chapel Hill Hospital to determine if the tumor had changed in size. My first MRI and scans were conducted at an imaging center about two miles from the hospital, and although I had been to multiple appointments at the main hospital, I didn't know just where the imaging center was located in the building. This MRI was scheduled for 6:45 on a Thursday night. I had been keeping my cancer appointments either before or after work, as we had not yet shared our diagnosis with many people.

I was beginning to realize that my almost picture-perfect life was getting ready to change and would become very difficult. It was just starting to hit me that what we were going through was serious and life threatening. That night would put things in perspective for me.

I checked in at the main desk and they informed me that the imaging center was just past the Children's Hospital, which was also on the hospital campus. I began the 10-minute walk but stopped about halfway there. I was looking into a room that was labeled as a parents' waiting room. About 25-30 adults were waiting on updates for their children who were either in surgery or recovering from surgery. Covid rules at that time only allowed one parent to visit with their child at a time on the hospital floors while the other family members had to wait in this designated waiting room on the first floor. You could see the nerves on each of their faces and I am sure many tears were cried in that room.

This walk was a defining moment for me. I would never allow myself to throw a pity party, asking why did cancer choose me. The courage and bravery shown by these children and their families fighting a similar fight as me far surpassed anything I could accomplish with my own treatment. I cannot imagine if my kids were going through what I have, and I have so much admiration and respect for parents whose children need constant clinical and medical attention. Tomorrow is not guaranteed for anyone, and these parents were doing their best to help get their children healed physically and emotionally and getting them home. I don't have it that bad. Perspective.

I was an awful leader for my first two leadership roles. I felt being a leader was about me and focused all my energies on tasks for my personal career advancement.

My perspectives and priorities were not focused on the right things. I ignored the most important part of leading a team, which is the shared success of exceeding a goal, and making sure your individual team members flourish and develop. I have hopefully improved my skillset of leading others since I was promoted to my first leadership role at the ripe age of 25. Yet I still learn something new every week, with 25 years of leading others shaping me into the leader I am today. Always Learning.

When I was in elementary school, I learned a valuable lesson from my dad on the way to visit his mom in New York City. It centered on the art of telling someone what they mean to you. It was around the time that Britain's Princess Diana had passed away. Elton John had reworked his song "Candle in the Wind" as a tribute to her, and it was playing on the car radio, #1 on Kasey Kasem's Top 40 countdown. I shared with my dad how impressed I was that he did that. My dad said "Sure, but she is no longer with us. I hope Elton John told her how important she was to him prior to her passing". I am not sure why, but this has stuck with me throughout my life. I remember the weather that day (cold, gray and damp) and we were under an overpass as we had just crossed the Triboro Bridge into Manhattan.

I need to tell the significant people in my life how important they are every day. This concept did not hit me until marriage, and never really took hold until I became a leader of others several years later. Never let people doubt how you feel about them. In our world, we get too caught up in the day-to-day tasks whether at home, school, sports, activities, etc. We are constantly "on", connected via text, email, phone, Snapchat, Instagram and many more apps and communication tools. We don't take the time to slow down and cherish what we have living in a wonderful country, with freedoms many times being taken for granted. You cannot run a marathon at a sprinter's pace or you will wear down and collapse from exhaustion. Establishing a productive pace at home and work is critical to mental well-being.

When I was diagnosed with cancer in March 2021, we had an outpouring of support for our family. As the news spread, friends, colleagues, and extended family members that we had not heard from or talked to in years offered their thoughts and prayers. We welcomed all these wonderful gestures of kindness. Christy and I slowly began to talk with these friends who we had met over the years, and family members we lost touch with. It should not have taken a tragedy to reconnect with these people who were involved with us at some point in our lives.

With this remembered perspective of connecting, I prioritized spending more time with our children. I travel a lot for my job, and am happy to do so. Typically, I would be gone Tuesday through Thursday. Over the years, I have missed games, school dances, and many other events while on the road, not to mention things like practices, homework, and after-school activities. These midweek days that I was on the road were also the times where I would notice multiple debits in our bank account for Chick-Fil-A and Bojangles, as my wife is allergic to cooking at home while I am out of town. Seriously, Christy ran the house and did a wonderful job keeping up with everything. Now that I was stuck at home in recovery for the next couple months, I prioritized to get healthy, fully recover, and build stronger relationships with Connor and Kelcie. We raised our children on the premise that they, as well as Christy and I, would make mistakes with family decisions. It's okay to make mistakes because that is where true growth comes from. We would learn from these missteps, not make the same mistake again, and move on.

Connor is a strong and unique leader both on the field and off. He may never be the smartest in the classroom or the best athlete on the field, but he loves the grind of getting things done. This desire to get better each week helped him earn soccer All-American status his senior year. He was the only goalkeeper to make this list, and was the first All-American in Wake Forest High School history.

He also loves to serve others, and helped organize and lead fundraisers to support Make-A-Wish Eastern NC and the Leukemia & Lymphoma Society, raising over $75,000 for these two charities while in high school. He can stand up in front of a room full of adults, say a heartwarming grace prior to a meal, then have mature conversations with these adults on multiple topics. I knew he was doing well and was ready to make the leap to college, but was shocked by how composed and confident he was. I was now witnessing the little things he accomplished during the week that were part of his grind to excel in games, schools and on weekends. He was now a man.

As stated earlier, Connor coined the phrase "We Got This" as our rallying cry for treatment. Never once did I see him cry or get emotional when he learned of my cancer diagnosis. He did that in the privacy of his room and with friends. I know he was hiding it from his sister, because he had to be the strong one, not showing her that he was upset or worried…like a good big brother should behave. If Kelcie saw Connor upset, then she would be upset as well. She looks up to her big brother.

I have two cherished documents that are the most important things in the world to me. One is my marriage license with Christy. The other is a letter Connor wrote for me that was in my suitcase the morning of my surgery. Over the years, I have hand-written letters to both my kids before a big game or big test, or if I was going to miss an event that was important to them. Putting these notes in their cleats, gloves, or backpacks, they would open them up when they arrived at the event to prepare, and hopefully gain some added motivation to perform well. Connor had given his letter to Christy before we left for Charleston. I was blown away by his courage and conviction. When I experience challenging days with pain, I go into my office and read the letter. I cry every time and it grounds me. Perspective.

My daughter Kelcie is turning into a startling young woman. She is freakishly athletic, with height and speed, and has a physical nature that follows her on the soccer field. She is known to frustrate opposing players with her style of play, typically "trucking" a player or two per game. One parent on an opposing team shouted at the referee "That girl is playing like a linebacker," as Kelcie physically overpowered one of their players. We exposed both of our kids to many different sports and activities in their elementary school days. We shared that they needed to love what they did outside of school, but they would be committed to some type of extracurricular activity in middle school and high school. Kelcie was great at everything she tried... swimming, gymnastics, dance, running track. Connor and Kelcie both chose soccer as the sport they love.

Kelcie is beautiful inside and out. Like any dad watching their baby girl turn into a young woman, I have a mini heart attack every time she comes down the steps dressed in a nice outfit to hang with friends. To me, every top she wears is too short and every skirt or dress needs to be longer. She is also strong-willed and stubborn, willing to challenge her mom and me on decisions we have made that she does not agree with. She provides data to us on why she needs the new pair of Lulu shorts or Nike shoes (sometimes this answer is yes if her grades are good and her room is organized), why we should change houses and move to Eastern Tennessee or to the beach (this answer is always no), or why we need to get another dog (a strong no to this weekly request).

Kelcie is learning how to grind in life, whether working hard at school, fighting through knee pain to not let her team down in soccer, or to be in the best shape possible for running and endurance. She played in two state cup games in May, just three weeks after her knee was scoped and debrided. Behind this exterior strength and hard-headedness is a sweet person, who truly cares about what people think of her and how she comes across. She is overly protective with me, making sure I am not lifting things that are too heavy or doing too much. She has a love for all animals, especially dogs, and talks a lot about being a veterinarian or running a shelter for rescue dogs as she gets older. She is self-sufficient at home, making her own lunches, doing her laundry, and we know how well our dogs are treated when she is in charge. She moves around furniture in her bedroom every month or so to try and view life differently from the confines of her room. She does not ask for our help with that, and has figured out how to use the right tools and things to help her slide beds and dressers on her own. She is learning how to be a better teammate, student, and friend. I have seen her mature so much in the last eight months to become more confident. She is going to be outstanding at anything she does.

We all have scars, both external and internal. Scars indicate pain and then healing. External scars are visible to all. Internal scars are hidden and are only released when a person chooses to do so. While I will bear the external scars on my head and back for the rest of my life, I cry when I think of the internal scars I have given Christy, Connor, and Kelcie. We tend to bottle up our frustration and hurt feelings, not wanting to show weakness or fault. We talk as a family a lot, asking our kids about what's on their mind. We have heard some brutal truths from them, and sometimes way too much information shared (TMI). We have had some very poignant and meaningful conversations around discussing our scars. We are all scarred from our fight with cancer but we are healing them as a team.

I share these words because of the life-work balance we all look to have. Some months have us tilting toward spending more time at work than with the important things in your personal life. Effective people and leaders will need to counterbalance that time spent so the life-work balance pendulum is always centered. Even though my work priorities had changed from working at Align to battling cancer, I tried to make sure my pendulum was balanced.

With the news from October 11th that we were in remission, our priority shifted to try and heal the wounds that were stalled on my head and back. For my back, we decided to treat this wound with a partial thickness skin graft. For this surgery, the surgeon would take a Dermatome (similar to a cheese grater) and slice a layer off my outer thigh, like cutting a slice from a block of cheese. The surgeon would then take the skin, which was a little bit bigger than an iPhone, stretch it out, and suture it onto my back. This was the most effective way to close that wound.

We again were re-introduced to my friend, the wound VAC. It was placed on my back for seven days to help the back wound heal. With skin grafts, I had always learned that the donor site would be more painful than the recipient site on my back. This was indeed the case. We had been asked to try a new type of pain management, a cutting-edge technology, for the donor site for this surgery. We were told this product would be less invasive to the wound and help alleviate pain in a more effective manner. After surgery, I was asked by my nurse what my pain level was for my donor site. She said it should be one or two out of 10, with little to no pain or discomfort. My pain level was nine out of 10. I told her to take this thing off my leg. I did not endorse this new product!

During this surgery, the surgeons also continued to work on the stubborn wounds on my forehead incision site. We still had three open areas on my head, on the front, side and back. The site which had opened during radiation in July was still causing problems. The surgeons pulled the forehead and flap on my head tighter together, stitched and stapled them and tried to get them to hold. While still open, we were getting a little closer to having skin touch skin in these troublesome wounds.

I was discharged the day after that operation. I still had not experienced a good night's sleep since late April, and another night in a hospital did not interest me at all. We made the 4.5-hour trip back to Wake Forest, listening to Dave Grohl read his best-selling book, Storytellers, to us over the radio. I hopped into the La-Z-Boy recliner that had been my place of refuge and some shuteye over the last seven months. I thought about our journey and how we had gotten to this point of remission, overcoming each obstacle thrown at us.

My answer was Christy. Prior to cancer, I tried to make sure Christy always knew my #1 priority was to make her smile and laugh, and I would love her until my dying day. I committed to recognizing her as much as possible so she knew how much I loved her, if anything bad were to happen to me: flowers, chocolate, hand-written notes, chocolate, little gifts from every trip I was on, and still more chocolate. She is a remarkable woman who I am fortunate to share life with. She is humble without being a pushover. She is genuine without trying to be so. She is kind and empathetic toward everyone she meets. She enables us all, but puts up boundaries to make sure we don't feel entitled. She asks for very little in life and is grateful for the things she has, not taking anything for granted. She under-promises and over-delivers in everything she does. She is the best human being I know. She did not have much growing up. When asking her grandfather for his blessing to marry Christy, I promised him that I would spoil her every day as this is what she deserved. I have been committed to never let her down and will never give up fighting cancer to stand by her side for the next 21 years and beyond.

After my cancer diagnosis, she took on the dual role of loving wife and caregiver with me, making me her top priority. I truly am in awe of how she has handled the medical part of helping me with dressing changes and cleaning out wounds, or administering antibiotics. I have joked with her that I cannot make her mad at any time during treatment. If I do, I know the tape on my back and my head will be removed with a certain force and speed during our daily dressing changes, which would cause me a lot of pain. "Ripping the bandage" would replace "gently removing the bandage" if I made her mad. She wields that power, but does not take advantage of it.

I got lucky with her. Perspective.

ALWAYS LEARNING LEADER TAKEAWAYS:

Life-work balance and mental health are essential topics today. While dealing with Covid, many people struggled with how to successfully understand this new world we were thrust into, and not prepared for. We learned on the fly, and while some people and companies prospered, many experienced challenges that will take them years to learn from and overcome. Some ideas for helping with this for professional and personal growth:

- At work, schedule meetings for 45-50 minutes instead of a full hour. Avoid having to run from one meeting to the next, as we see happen when a one-hour meeting runs long. You have to sprint to the next meeting, stressing about your tardiness. This "interval" type of approach with a quick break between meetings is something I find makes people more efficient when we are talking business.

- Also at work, block out a 30-60-minute period per day to get caught up on email, administrative work, callbacks, etc. Something outside of a meeting with a set agenda with others. Walk around the office or take a quick five to 10-minute walk outside.

- For personal growth, set a weekly appointment with yourself for 30-45 minutes to listen to a podcast or read a professional or personal development book. Treat this time as if it was an appointment with your most important customer. If a work commitment gets scheduled at the same time, then move your personal development time to another available slot in your calendar. My personal development time is 7:30am-8:00am every Friday. No calls, no texts, no emails.

VIEW THE PICTURES THAT
CHRONICLE OUR JOURNEY

ALWAYSLEARNINGLEADER.COM/WE-GOT-THIS-PICTURES/

CHAPTER 8

Reaching Goals
& No Finish Line
*NOVEMBER 2021 – JANUARY 2022

We have talked a lot about self-improvement, and to always be learning in our lives. As leaders and team members, we have to constantly work on our skillsets as well as learn from others about how they are successful. I would also share that we learn a lot from the "not-so-good" leaders in our lives about what not to do in certain situations. Some of my best takeaways are the result of learning from others' successes and mistakes. There should be no finish line when it comes to how you develop in life.

We have learned that there is no finish line with cancer. The surgeries and procedures we encountered in 2021 all presented us with benefits and risks. We also know that many of the risks, while not present in my body now, can turn up again without warning. Reoccurrence is common for the cancer I have (67% in two years).

Side effects from radiation remain in your body for three to five years past your last treatment. Skin cancers will reappear in other parts of my body, many of which have not seen the light of day since high school. While wounds will be healed, the skin never gains back 100% of its tensile strength and can be re-opened if too much is done too soon.

While we searched for the new normal for our family and for me, we realized in November that it will never again be constant. The new normal we would experience in the coming years would be a regularly evolving journey between good days and challenging days. We needed to still get through each week, and not look too far into the future.

I have committed to the concept of "Post-Traumatic Growth" in my future, both personally and professionally. That means an individual who has suffered a traumatic experience somehow finds ways to turn it into something good. Typically, interpersonal relationships are improved, with friends and family valued more, and more time being spent in helping others.

I will never recover to be the exact version I was prior to 2021. However, I am now dedicated to being a better father, husband, friend, and leader than I was before our cancer diagnosis. I will have to work harder than ever to achieve these goals, and having the right support system around me to help both my physical and mental states will be important.

I love the book "Multipliers" by Liz Wiseman. This a required read for anyone in a leadership role working for me. The concept is simply stated below.

> *There are two types of leaders:*
>
> *The first type, **Diminishers**, drains intelligence, energy, and capability from the people around them and always needs to be the smartest person in the room.*
>
> *The second type, **Multipliers**, are the leaders who use their intelligence to amplify the smarts and capabilities of the people around them. When these leaders walk into a room, light bulbs go off over people's heads; ideas flow and problems get solved.*

After reading her book, and having everyone around me do so, we began to use the concept in our weekly meetings and we became more efficient. I also had family members read the book. My wife, again the leader in our household, would call me out as being a diminisher if my comments at home were negative or ill-guided toward my family. Cancer has made me irritable at times as I get frustrated with the physical recovery I am going through, and I must be better with handling this emotion.

There will always be naysayers, diminishers who feel they need to be the smartest person in the room. These leaders have made up their mind on what they think is right before gathering input and data from their team. This closed-off leadership style stunts individual and team growth, and will only create future followers and not develop future leaders.

Being a multiplier in a Post-Traumatic Growth scenario is going to be a challenge, but will be so rewarding. Simple tasks like getting dressed in the morning, taking a shower, preparing a meal all now take me two or three times longer than before surgery. My typing accuracy is now atrocious as my mind is working faster than my fingers can hit the keyboard. Every now and then, I get uncontrollable tremors in my fingers, causing the typing to be even worse. And while I feel my mind and memory are still sharp 95% of the time, there are times I struggle to think through a situation or problem. At times, I get frustrated with the way my mind and body communicate. However, my purpose is to continue to be a multiplier with the people around me. I just need to adapt my processes and planning with everything I do. Compared to our life prior to cancer, I will be a better multiplier now because of our cancer battle and the adversity we have overcome together.

Healthwise, as we approached Thanksgiving, the skin graft wounds on my back and thigh donor site wound were progressing as expected and we shifted our priorities to my three head wounds which were still struggling to heal. Two of the wounds now had exposed hardware. This was going to be the next challenge for us in getting completely healed.

We drove back to MUSC in Charleston on November 22nd for another CT scan and a PET scan to prepare us for surgery the second week of December. The PET scan is an interesting procedure lasting about 60-90 minutes in total treatment time. The nurses begin by injecting a dye into the IV in your arm, which you can feel slowly move throughout your body with a warm sensation. After the dye is injected, we wait about five minutes, and dim all the lights in the room. The nurses leave me alone in the semi-dark room and I then have to sit for 60 minutes in complete silence, without noise, or access to music, text messages, emails, TV, etc. Just me, my thoughts, and a room...for an hour. It's crazy what you think about during these hour-long sessions.

When the hour of quiet time is up, we move to the PET scan room and I am placed on another flat board. The PET scan machine slowly and methodically scans my entire body, looking for any signs of cancer or other abnormalities. This is a very comprehensive scan of my body, and will help us determine the next steps for surgery and if the cancer is back. The good news is both scans revealed no signs of the cancer in my body.

We now began the discussions with our surgical team on my three head wounds. December was also the month where we would try and re-shape my head back to normal from its current rhombus shape. I did not want to have two different surgeries done in December. Our surgical team felt confident that they could close all three wounds and re-shape my head in one surgery, but the exposed hardware in two of the wounds was a concern. We could see the aqua colored titanium plate in those wounds, which is not good. Sometimes a foreign object like hardware such as a titanium plate for the head, hip replacement or knee replacement is rejected by the body and needs to be removed and replaced. Our specific negative situation was likely caused by the infections in my head from August, and the doctors felt that the plate was now colonized with infection.

The surgeons could not commit to how they would treat this operation as it could vary depending on what they would find. They may have to remove the flap from my head, remove parts of the titanium plate or even the entire plate from my head, put a new plate in, and hope the existing flap is still intact and the right size to place over the new plate in my head. If not, we will have to take a new flap from somewhere else in my body, and I will be one of the few people to have two full-thickness skin flaps on my head. Surgery could last anywhere from four to 10 hours, depending on what they find when they begin the procedure. While these meetings provided us challenging information to process, we felt confident in the plan. WE GOT THIS!!!

Surgery was scheduled for December 14th in Charleston. While we were all hoping for the shorter and simpler four-hour surgery, we prepared as though we were going to endure the more complex 10-hour option. I began working on my physical endurance to support my mental endurance. I started doing longer walks as part of my physical therapy, and even got back on the Peloton for some 20–30-minute rides. I was convinced that my body and mind would be ready to crush this next surgery.

We were able to spend time with our family at Thanksgiving. We hosted my brother, my sister and her family, and my mom for the afternoon. I am really close to my mom, and while we don't see her as often as we would like, we talk three to four times per week. She was the rock for my dad while he battled pancreatic cancer. Before I found out I had cancer, she would often cry or get emotional about something going on in her life, such as a friend passing away or learning of someone who is not doing well, or even just little things like stressing about the state of our world. She has always been a worrier. She wears her emotions on her sleeve. Now that we are fighting cancer, I think she cries when she sees me, cries a couple of times per phone call, and cries when we hang up. When my dad passed away from his cancer, I made a promise to him that I would look after and take care of my mom. She is a special woman and I am confident she knows how I feel about her.

Sunday, December 10th started off as a great day. Connor had just finished final exams the day before, and was going to be home for the next 40 days. Christy was intent on giving him special mom hugs, which typically every child tries to avoid. These hugs were shared pretty much each time she saw him in our home. She had set a goal of giving him five to 10 of these hugs per day.

Sunday night we started to pack for our trip to Charleston, knowing we could be there for three days to recover, or it could be seven days if the surgery was the more complex version. Christy packed her workout clothing along with her sweats for the hospital. We always tried to stay at a hotel with a Peloton in the gym. Riding the Peloton was where Christy went when she needed healing. So many rides, thoughts, tears, and comfort were found on the seat of that bike for her. I packed underwear and t-shirts to wear underneath my surgical gown post-surgery.

I came downstairs at 7:45pm after she changed the wound dressings on my head. A new episode of Yellowstone was coming on at 8:00, and we were excited to watch this week's event. While Christy was finishing packing in our bedroom, she heard a disturbing wheezing, grunting, and rustling sound downstairs. At first, she thought it was our dogs playing, but she ran down the stairs to find me unresponsive on our sectional sofa. While she was talking to me, I was unconscious and convulsing, leaned over at a very uncomfortable angle. She said my eyes were rolling up back under my eyelids, and the sound coming out of my mouth was just babbling. There was blood and drool near my mouth, which we would later learn came from me biting my tongue during this episode. I heard her talking to me but could not respond. I had no idea what was happening, and had no control over anything on my body.

She called 911 and my blood pressure had ballooned to 250/165 when the EMS team arrived. They put us in the ambulance and we once again made the 45-minute drive to the UNC Hospital emergency room. The emergency room was very crowded on this Sunday night, and in the first 20 minutes in the ER, I had three different nurses unsuccessfully try to insert an IV into my arms. I continued to be a tough stick with needles. We met with our nurses and doctors quickly after registration and everyone confirmed that all signs pointed to me having a seizure, which is a common side effect after radiation. My heart rate had slowed down to normal levels in the ambulance ride over. They needed to run some tests to determine if I had any neurological damage from the seizure, and hopefully avoid another one occurring. The neurologist told us that for this type of seizure and for patients that went through similar radiation protocols, one out of every three patients would have a second seizure within five days. The doctors prescribed me an antiseizure medicine to start immediately.

This seizure two days before our head wound surgery would cause us to reschedule with our surgeons in Charleston for January as my body was not able to handle another traumatic event in a 48-hour period. Due to NC driving laws, I would not be able to drive a car for six months. We were discharged and got home at 5:30 Monday morning. We would try to schedule some tests, including another MRI, in the next 48 hours.

Tuesday morning had us back in the hospital to have another MRI performed. This time we were at Wake Med in Raleigh, as their imaging center was the first one we could get into. After an hour in the MRI machine, I returned to our room awaiting the results.

These few days had us listening to different interpretations of all these new scans from doctors who were new to us and our case. I was trying to talk normally again but this took a while due to my swollen tongue. My mind was also not working as quickly as it was prior to surgery and these delays in speech and reactions were concerning. At Wake Med, our P.A. told us he believed the MRI showed that the cancer was back, and through the dura layer into my brain. After he shared this news with us, he left the room, and both Christy and I lost it, crying uncontrollably. We know that our cancer is going to come back at some point and I will eventually not be able to overcome the effects cancer has on my body, but we were just cleared three weeks ago with no signs of cancer. However, after remembering our journey finding out about Porocarcinoma, and how fast this disease spreads and grows, it was not surprising that this could be a possibility. We wanted another opinion or two from doctors who were more intimately involved with our case and my head.

We sent the MRI images to both Dr. Day in Charleston and Dr. Rauf at UNC-Chapel Hill. We met with Dr. Rauf and she informed us that even though the MRI showed a new small mass on the brain, it was not necessarily cancer. It could have been a result from the seizure or something else entirely. She left open the possibility of conducting a needle biopsy during the reconstructive surgery in Charleston. Chemotherapy was still not an option, but depending on what the surgeons found during surgery, another series of radiation treatments could be in my future.

Dr. Day confirmed what Dr. Rauf shared and we rescheduled surgery for January 4th. We were able to spend Christmas Day together as a family, and even went to the beach for three days. It was a great week for our family, in spite of the seizure I had just experienced two weeks ago.

On Monday, January 3rd, Christy and I once again made the 4.5-hour drive to Charleston. We met with the surgical team to discuss what would be our fifth open-head surgery in nine months, and hopefully our last for a while. Our surgeons were optimistic but also shared that we were now getting to a point that my head could not be opened too many more times to try to close the wounds. There was a chance I could have open wounds on my head for the rest of my life, covered with bandages. Also, the new Omicron variant was having an impact on rules for hospital visitors and Christy would only be able to see me from 10:00am to 6:00pm each day.

Christy dropped me off at the surgery center on Tuesday, January 4th at 5:30am. Surgery started around 8:00am and we were finished around 4:30pm. The surgeons all said the surgery was a success in getting the wounds closed and there were no signs of cancer from the needle biopsies performed. They replaced a part of the titanium plate in my head that had come loose. That was great news. It was only one part, and not the whole plate they had to fix. They also told us the recovery from this surgery was going to be painful due to the stretching and pulling of my skin to get the wounds closed. I would spend the next three weeks having my wounds cleaned and dressed twice per day. There would be no physical activity allowed as we did not want to put any strain or stress on these sutured and stapled areas on my head, and I would basically be confined to my recliner and bed. But we were getting closer to healing. I was discharged two days after surgery on January 6th, and made it home for my son's 19th birthday dinner.

It is tough to run a race or work on a project that does not have a true finish line. The importance of setting small realistic goals and developing processes around them is more critical than ever. My short-term goals are the following:

1. Wake up pain-free and wound-free for the first time since April 26, 2021. Physical therapy and surgery will help with this.
2. Make it to the next holiday on our calendar. Birthdays and anniversaries count for this as well.
3. Return to work as quickly as possible.
4. Send 25 recognition text messages, emails or phone calls each week.
5. One Family Gratitude text per day from me to Christy, Connor and Kelcie. Giving thanks and showing gratitude should not be limited to certain holidays. We were going to be better as a family.

ALWAYS LEARNING LEADER TAKEAWAYS:

- Be a Fountain vs. a Drain – I love this analogy for how comments in a meeting or in conversations are perceived. I also use this same rule for social media to determine if a person is a fountain or drain. I prefer to be a fountain, providing positive flow with work, friends and family. I am far from 100% perfect on this, but I do catch myself when I am making draining comments.

- Four Important Rules of Growth (modified from a post from Peloton instructor Kendall Toole, Christy's and my favorite instructor):

  a. Speak Less

     i. Focus on purpose and process and your results will speak for you.

  b. Listen More

     i. Make sure to practice your listening skills, such as reflection.

     ii. Don't interrupt...no matter how hard it is.

  c. Observe More

     i. The more you observe, the clearer the situation.

     ii. The clearer the situation, the better your reaction.

     iii. The better your reaction, the better your results.

d. React Less

    i. Emotional Intelligence is so important.

    ii. The less you react, the better you will respond.

VIEW THE PICTURES THAT
CHRONICLE OUR JOURNEY

ALWAYSLEARNINGLEADER.COM/WE-GOT-THIS-PICTURES/

PARTING WORDS

As stated in Chapter 8, there is no finish line for surviving cancer and for personal and professional development. As individuals and businesses, we are either shrinking or growing. Very rarely will there be a constant neutral state and if there is, then both companies and individuals will grow stagnant and get passed by. I hope sharing our 12-month cancer story over these eight chapters instilled some inspiration and belief in overcoming anything thrown in your way in life, while positively impacting others. I hope it made you "Think, Laugh, and Cry" at some point. I also hope that it challenged you to think about your legacy, and your impact on others. To me, my legacy will not be determined by the things I leave behind, but in the hearts and lives that I have had a positive impression on.

I wrote this book to share our journey through 2021 (and wound up going into January 2022). We are hopeful that 2022 will be a better year for all of us. To again quote the legendary Jimmy Valvano, "Cancer can take away all of my physical abilities. It cannot touch my mind, it cannot touch my heart, and it cannot touch my soul."

One out of four people will be stricken with some type of cancer in their lifetime. Feel free to e-mail me at jfkitson@gmail.com if you have someone you know who is struggling with cancer and its side effects and I will be there to listen. I will also resume my quarterly blog at www.alwayslearningleader.com in 2022 and update pictures using the link and QR code contained in this book.

We are blessed to be living our version of "The New Normal" and I plan on kicking cancer's ass for many years to come.

WE GOT THIS!

Jimmy

Made in United States
North Haven, CT
15 July 2022